making babies

The New Zealand Guide to Getting Pregnant
Edited by Dr Mary Birdsall

FERTILITY ASSOCIATES
New Edition

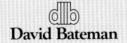

David Bateman

First published in 2009 by David Bateman Ltd,
30 Tarndale Grove, Albany, Auckland, New Zealand

www.batemanpublishing.co.nz

Reprinted 2012

ISBN 978-1-86953-711-1

Book design and typesetting: Alice Bell
Cover images: front — Getty Images; back — iStock
Printed in China by Everbest Printing Co. Ltd

Contents

About Fertility Associates

Pioneering reproductive medicine in New Zealand, Fertility Associates was first established in Auckland in 1987. Co-founders Dr Richard Fisher and Dr Freddie Graham were both previously responsible for introducing in vitro fertilisation (IVF) technology to New Zealand in 1983, where they ran a fertility clinic at the original National Women's Hospital in Auckland.

As New Zealand's leading provider of fertility diagnosis, support and treatment, Fertility Associates have been busy building families for over 20 years — with over 8500 babies born to date. Committed to excellence and integrity, each Fertility Associates clinic has a close-knit team of doctors, nurses, counsellors and scientists dedicated to providing optimum care and giving you the best possible chance of having a baby.

Offering private and publicly funded consultation and treatment, Fertility Associates is active in both community and professional education and undertakes a number of research programmes.

Fertility Associates have three main clinics located in Auckland, Hamilton and Wellington which feature modern, comfortable facilities and state-of-the-art equipment and technology. We also have a number of satellite clinics located around the country including Auckland's North Shore, Whangarei, Tauranga, Rotorua, Hawke's Bay, Gisborne, New Plymouth, Palmerston North and Nelson.

We offer a full range of services, from the most simple to the most advanced technology available worldwide. We provide a full range of counselling services including decision-making and support during assessment and treatment. We also offer lifestyle programmes including weight-loss and exercise.

If you have a fertility question that remains unanswered, the sooner you talk to us, the better your chances of having a baby. When it comes to fertility, we understand.

Introduction

The desire to have a family is, for most of us, a strong one, and being unable to fulfil that basic need is enormously traumatic. *Making Babies* has been written to provide you with some understanding of fertility. This updated edition includes recent advances in IVF, lifestyle advice and current thinking about all aspects of infertility.

The physiological processes involved in reproduction are overviewed along with some advice on how to look after your fertility. Many people spend years avoiding pregnancy and then wish to become pregnant and we therefore discuss how to maximise your chances.

The book then concentrates on what to do if a pregnancy is not occurring, when to get worried, where to seek help, what tests will be done and the treatment options available. A chapter on endometriosis is included because this is a common problem which is often poorly managed, leading to fertility problems later on. We have added a new chapter on sperm problems, as sperm issues may be increasing in frequency.

We have also included a chapter on what to do when pregnancy does occur and potential problems in early pregnancy. A chapter on coping with the stress of infertility has been written by the counsellors at Fertility Associates. We have also included a list of support and information groups and societies in New Zealand.

We hope this book enhances your understanding of fertility and helps you have a baby.

Fertility Associates, 2009

Authors:
Mary Birdsall
Joi Ellis
Richard Fisher
Freddie Graham
John Peek

CHAPTER ONE

HOW TO BECOME PREGNANT

When is the right time to have a baby? Only you will know the answer, but in making the decision to try for a baby, there are many factors to consider that will influence your chances of conception. This chapter discusses the biological and lifestyle issues that will help and inform you.

What happens when you stop contraception?

The first thing to do when you have decided to try for a baby is to stop contraception. If you are using a barrier method such as condoms or a diaphragm, obviously you can just stop using it. If you have been using an intrauterine contraceptive device (IUCD) you need to have this removed by your doctor, which can be done with a minimal amount of discomfort in your doctor's surgery.

The oral contraceptive pill (oestrogen progesterone combination) prevents you having normal periods and as soon as you stop taking it your periods will return. There is no evidence that the pill causes infertility, and 80% of women who stop the pill will become pregnant over the next year, which is the same as for women who are not taking the pill. You may even conceive immediately after stopping the pill.

Depo-Provera injections (progesterone only) also stop normal periods but will delay the return of normal periods by at least five months after the last injection, so you need to plan ahead if you have been using this form of contraception.

Sex and conception

An enjoyable sex life is an important part of a happy relationship but some couples find that the fun and spontaneity are lost whilst they try for a baby, especially if they don't conceive within the first few months. Many myths surround sex for conception so let's dispel those and focus on what you need to do to become pregnant.

When to have sex

The window of opportunity is small and therefore it is important to get the timing right. Sex one or two days before ovulation is the most likely time to result in pregnancy, as sperm can survive in the female reproductive tract for around three days, but the egg must be fertilised within 18–24 hours of ovulation. If you have sex the day after ovulation it is less likely to result in pregnancy. For most women, ovulation occurs two weeks before the start of the next period, which is around day 14 of a 28-day cycle. However, all women are different and a normal cycle can vary, so it is important to know your own cycle.

How often to have sex

You cannot have sex too often when you are trying to conceive, so the more the better. Many ejaculations in a short space of time do not 'weaken' the sperm, in fact sperm quality improves with frequent ejaculation, therefore saving up sperm for a particular day will not increase your chances of success. There is some evidence that ovulation usually happens in daylight hours, so an afternoon off once a month may be more effective than a romantic evening.

How to have sex

No sexual position has been found to be better for conception, so just do what feels right for you as a couple as long as the man's sperm ejaculates directly into the woman's vagina. Female orgasm may improve tubal motility, but there is no evidence that it improves the chances of conception. Lying with your pillow under your bottom or legs up the wall does not improve the chances of pregnancy and it is also OK to pass urine after sex.

Predicting your fertile time

Having a regular menstrual cycle, which is defined as one period every 25 to 35 days with a less than four-day variation between cycles, may help you to predict when you are about to ovulate without resorting to any form of test. Here are some prediction tips:

• **Abdominal pain or discomfort:** Many women can actually feel when they ovulate because of this 'mittelschmerz' or middle month pain.

• **Mucus changes:** Cervical mucus is usually thick and sticky to prevent infection by invading bacteria. However, when oestrogen levels are high and ovulation is imminent, it changes in consistency to become clear and fluid (like egg white), which allows sperm to swim through more easily and this is the best time for sex.

• **Luteinising hormone kits:** These detect the concentration of luteinising hormone in your urine. The levels of this hormone rise sharply just before ovulation but this increase only lasts for around 24–36 hours, so the best time to have sex is within 24 hours of testing positive. Be wary of false positives that can happen due to some hormonal conditions, such as polycystic ovaries. These kits can be purchased off the internet or from a pharmacy.

• **Temperature charts:** Ovulation coincides with an increase in body temperature of 0.5 to 1.6°C, but as the most fertile time is just before peak temperature increase, this is not helpful for timing when to have sex, but may help to establish a pattern for prediction. This is not the most useful method as temperature charts are frequently misleading and are a constant reminder that you are trying to conceive.

• **Blood test:** The most reliable test to detect whether ovulation has occurred is a blood test to measure progesterone levels, which rise one week before the next period is due.

Don't wait too long

Age is a significant factor in fertility and is the most common reason for visits to a fertility clinic. On average it takes three to four months for a 25-year-old woman to conceive if everything else is

AGE	CHANCE OF CONCEIVING PER MONTH %
25	25%
30	20%
35	16%
37	11%
40	6%
42	4%
44	2%
45 and over	<2%

Table 1: Chance of conceiving each month according to a woman's age.

normal but it takes twice as long at age 35.

Chances of conception per month decrease significantly with increasing age and the time to conceive lengthens as age increases, even for normally fertile couples (see Table 1).

There is little difference up to about age 34, but from 35 years onwards there is a significant drop in the chance of conception per month and many couples find that they take much longer to conceive than they would like. By the time a woman reaches the age of 39 it is not uncommon for normally fertile couples to take more than 15 months to conceive, so the best advice to be offered is not to wait too long. The dilemma with increasing age is that biology severely limits the chance of conception per month when the need to conceive quickly is at its greatest. It is much more likely that a woman in her twenties has a significant problem if she has not conceived after six months of trying than a woman aged 37 who has not conceived after 15 months.

Men are also affected by increasing age, with a reduction in sperm quality along with a slightly increased risk of inherited conditions such as schizophrenia and dwarfism in children conceived by 'older' dads. The underlying mechanism is thought to be due to spontaneous mutations in the father's DNA.

Preconception care

There are some lifestyle changes you should consider, which will improve your chances of conceiving and having a healthy baby.

Folic acid and multivitamins

There is good evidence that folic acid reduces the chances of having a baby with spina bifida (when the spine does not develop normally). The recommended dose is 0.8 mg of folic acid daily for two months before conceiving and until 12 weeks of pregnancy. The major folic acid supplements in the New Zealand market include Elevit and Blackmores (Blackmores Pregnancy and Breast Feeding Gold, and Blackmores Conceive Well). Folic acid supplements that contain general multivitamins may also reduce the chances of cardiac, urinary and cleft lip abnormalities in babies. Vitamin A formulations should be avoided as they are linked with birth defects.

Stop smoking

Cigarettes have a huge impact on fertility. Women who smoke are only 60% as likely to conceive as non-smokers and smoking is also associated with miscarriage, small babies and earlier menopause. Smoking appears to speed up the reproductive clock sometimes by up to 10 years. Men who smoke have lower sperm counts and more malformed sperm than non-smokers and are more likely to have children who develop childhood cancer. Smoking marijuana is also thought to have a detrimental influence on sperm. The good news is that smoking-induced damage to fertility may be reversible. Sperm take around 72 days to fully form, so if you give up smoking at least three months before trying to conceive, sperm quality should improve.

Women should not smoke for at least three months before trying to conceive, as this is how long it takes for an egg to grow and mature. Nicotine patches may cause the same problems as smoking so should also be avoided.

Give up alcohol

Most people are aware of the detrimental effects that alcohol can have on a pregnancy, by causing fetal alcohol syndrome. However, moderate drinking whilst trying to conceive also reduces fertility. Research has shown that women drinking five units or less a week are twice as likely to conceive as women drinking 10 or more units. If there is a safe level of alcohol in pregnancy, it is not known, so it is better not to drink at all as soon as you know you are pregnant, preferably before.

Alcohol also affects testicular and sexual functioning in men, so large amounts of alcohol should be avoided. The current recommendation is that men should drink less than 20 units of alcohol per week. One unit of alcohol is defined as 8 g of ethanol and is equivalent to a small can of beer or a small glass of wine (125 ml).

Drink less caffeine

Caffeine intake can affect fertility in women, as it is associated with a longer time to conceive and also reduced chances of becoming pregnant on an in vitro fertilisation (IVF) programme. More than six cups of coffee a day may also be linked with miscarriage. Caffeine is not only contained in coffee but also in a variety of other products such as tea, cola, energy drinks, some frozen desserts and chocolate; so be aware of your overall caffeine intake. Male fertility does not appear to be affected by caffeine.

Avoid sexually transmitted infections (STIs)

The rates of STIs are increasing in New Zealand. Often, these infections cause few, if any, symptoms, so the damage they cause can go unnoticed until a couple tries to conceive. For example, there is approximately a 10% chance of one episode of chlamydia (a sexually transmitted bacterial infection) causing infertility in women.

The damage caused by STIs includes blocked Fallopian tubes, pelvic pain, ectopic pregnancy as well as male infertility. Condoms

CASE HISTORY

Lauren had four boyfriends whilst she was at university and used a number of contraceptive methods ranging from withdrawal to the pill or condoms. She married Michael at age 26 and they decided to have a family when she was 29. They were not too concerned that Lauren did not become pregnant after the first year of trying but as the second year rolled by they decided to seek help.

A laparoscopy revealed bilateral blocked swollen tubes called hydrosalpinges. This was probably caused by a previous tubal infection, although Lauren felt she had never been promiscuous and had never had any symptoms of pelvic infection. Her tubes were too badly scarred for repair by surgery and so IVF was their only option. Before IVF, her damaged tubes were removed as this improves chances of pregnancy using IVF in women who have had some types of tubal damage. They conceived on their first IVF cycle and still have five frozen embryos.

should be used in all new sexual relationships to avoid risk of infection.

Maintain a healthy body weight

Being overweight or underweight can reduce fertility, so it is important to keep your body weight within the normal healthy range. Body Mass Index (BMI) is an indication of your body weight and can be calculated by dividing weight (in kg) by height (in m^2) (see Figure 1). You should aim for a BMI of between 20 and 25, as this will optimise your chances of conception.

Even in these modern times, nature knows best. If a woman's BMI falls below 19, the body senses famine and ovulation is switched off to prevent the risk of having a baby with malnutrition. Excessive

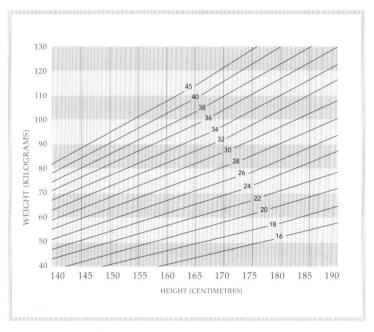

Figure 1: Body mass index (BMI) chart.
Each diagonal line represents the BMI in kg/m².

exercise can reduce body fat and increase muscle mass to a point where periods cease for the same reason. Risk of miscarriage is also increased in women with a low BMI.

Being overweight (BMI>30) can reduce fertility by 50%. Pregnancy in overweight women is often associated with problems such as maternal diabetes, high blood pressure, big babies and increased risk of caesarean section.

The good news is, however, that as soon as you get back on track with your body weight, ovulation and fertility quickly return to normal. Even a minimal weight loss (less than 5% of body weight) can make a difference, therefore advice with weight and its management is an important part of fertility treatment.

In men, being slightly overweight may also reduce sperm count, so men should also make an effort to keep their BMI within the normal range.

Reduce stress

Couples experiencing infertility definitely experience considerable stress, but whether stress causes infertility is a much debated issue, but one effect it can have is to interrupt a normal sex life resulting in less frequent sex. Extreme stress can switch off ovulation completely; however, cognitive therapy can help to reduce stress and has been shown to restart ovulation.

There is also some evidence that women who are clinically depressed when they start an IVF cycle are less likely to conceive. So our take home message is to look after yourself and your relationship by managing stress and seeking help if needed. You can read more about how to cope with the stress of infertility in Chapter 10.

What should you eat?

The current dietary advice is to eat a healthy balanced diet with lots of fresh fruit and vegetables. There are no wonder foods that will boost fertility, however there are some foods you could eat more of and others to be avoided. For men, there are a number of studies suggesting that antioxidants such as vitamin C and E, along with zinc and selenium may reduce DNA damage in sperm. Foods rich in antioxidants are good for both prospective parents, and include:

- all types of berries
- fruits such as grapes, oranges, plums, pineapple, dates, kiwifruit, mandarins
- dried fruit such as apricots and prunes
- vegetables such as red cabbage, peppers, parsley, artichokes, Brussels sprouts, tomatoes, spinach; brightly coloured vegetables are particularly rich in antioxidants

- legumes such as broad beans, groundnuts, soybeans
- cereals such as barley, millet, oats and corn
- nuts and seeds such as walnuts, brazil nuts, sunflower seeds
- garlic and ginger
- dark chocolate

For women, there are some foods that should not be eaten frequently, such as some fish which may be high in mercury. The highest levels of mercury are found in shark, swordfish and marlin, with much lower levels in tuna.

A recent study also found that a diet containing high levels of 'transfats' doubled the chances of infertility in women. Transfats are formed when liquid oils are chemically treated to increase their shelf life (hydrogenation) and are present in a wide variety of foods, particularly in snack foods, biscuits and some takeaways.

Although an 'organic' diet is a healthy option, there is no evidence that it improves fertility.

Keep active

There is a surprising lack of data on the effect of exercise on fertility. However, moderate exercise is always a healthy option and should be encouraged. Excessive exercise may not be so beneficial, as it may switch off ovulation resulting in irregular or absent periods. Cutting back to moderate exercise may restore the normal menstrual cycle and hence fertility. We do not fully understand why ovulation ceases with regular strenuous exercise or a low body weight, but it may be explained by the complex interactions between body fat, brain chemicals and ovaries. Moderation is the key to exercise when trying to conceive. For men, even less is known about the effects of exercise and sperm. Male obesity is associated with lower sperm counts so again moderate exercise is the healthy and most beneficial approach.

CASE HISTORY

Lisa had severe anorexia at age 16 and did not have periods for three years. At the age of 29 she had a body mass index of 19. She was having about three periods a year and wished to become pregnant. Her eating disorder was under control but she still exercised for one to two hours per day. She was very resistant to decreasing her exercise programme but after persistent advice she cut down to 20 minutes per day. Over the next six months her weight increased by three kilograms and she conceived spontaneously.

What about medication?

It is wise to check with your doctor regarding any medication that you are both on, as there may be a better alternative while you are planning a pregnancy. For example, women taking medication for epilepsy or depression should discuss options with a medical practitioner. There are also some drugs which you may have taken in the past that may impact on fertility, particularly chemotherapy drugs.

CHAPTER TWO

HOW DOES MAKING BABIES WORK?

The physiology of human reproduction is explained in this chapter and will help you understand how the male and female parts work together to make a baby.

Female reproductive system

Ovaries and eggs

A woman's eggs are contained in her two ovaries, which are whitish structures about the size of a small golf ball. When a mature egg is released by the ovary (ovulation) it is picked up by the Fallopian tube, which is a thin tube about 10 cm long, running out from the uterus towards the ovary. The tubes are lined by fine hair-like structures called cilia, which help transport sperm and egg along the tubes and also waft the embryo into the uterus. The uterus, or womb, is shaped like an upside-down pear and is usually around 8–9 cm long. This is where the fetus is nurtured and nourished until it is fully developed into a baby. The entrance of the uterus is called the cervix and is located at the top of the vagina.

Eggs are present in a female baby from a few weeks after conception. A hundred or so cells migrate from the yolk sac of the fertilised egg, into the tiny fetus, and take up residence in the tissue on top of the kidney. In a fetus destined to become a girl this tissue turns into the ovary, and the migrating cells into eggs. These eggs multiply, so that by the sixth month of pregnancy there are about seven million. However, by the time a baby girl is born the number of eggs will already have fallen to about two million, and by puberty — the time her periods start — there will be just a few hundred thousand eggs remaining to last throughout her fertile years.

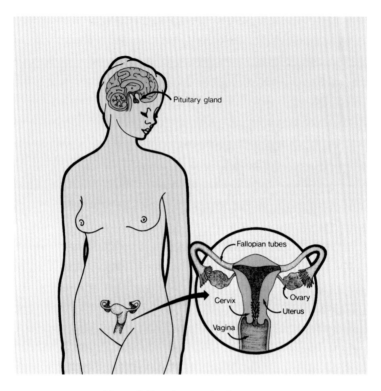

Figure 2: Female reproductive system.

Menstrual cycle

After puberty, the increasing levels of female reproductive hormones (oestrogen and progesterone) allow some of the eggs to mature and the menstrual cycle begins. The onset of periods (menarche) is a sign that the body is capable of sustaining a pregnancy. In the last three centuries in Western Europe, improved nutrition has lowered the average age of menarche from about 16 years of age to about 12 to 13. Today we consider it the norm for the menstrual cycle to begin in the early teens and last into the late forties. However, until recently, most of a woman's reproductive span was spent either pregnant or breastfeeding, and the number of menstrual cycles was many fewer than the 400 or so experienced by the 'modern' Western woman during her lifetime.

How does the menstrual cycle work?

• **Day 1:** Like all cycles, there is no real beginning or end to the menstrual cycle, but it is conventional to call the first day of bleeding Day 1.

• **The follicular stage:** The menstrual cycle is driven by the interaction of hormones from the brain and ovaries. The pituitary gland at the base of the brain begins to secrete follicle stimulating hormone (FSH) and luteinising hormone (LH). FSH stimulates eggs to mature within a fluid-filled structure called a follicle. The follicle is surrounded by granulosa cells, which provide the egg with nutrients and produce the hormone oestrogen. As the follicles grow, the number of granulosa cells increases and thus more oestrogen is produced. Each month about five to 15 follicles start to mature but usually only one will become dominant and develop fully to release an egg at ovulation. Ten to 14 days into the cycle the leading follicle will have grown from less than 5 mm in diameter to 20–25 mm. At this stage a mature follicle can easily be seen using ultrasound scanning, because it is filled with fluid. This first half of the menstrual cycle is called the follicular phase because it is dominated by what the follicles are doing. During this phase the lining of the uterus (endometrium) gradually increases in thickness to about 10–12 mm, which can also be seen by ultrasound scanning. The increasing levels of oestrogen from the granulosa cells promote endometrial growth.

• **Mid-cycle (ovulation):** When the egg is fully mature (about halfway through a menstrual cycle) the rising level of oestrogen in the blood stimulates the hypothalamus (a control centre in the brain) to send a message to the pituitary gland to release LH. This stimulates the follicle to burst open and release the egg. The event of ovulation defines the middle of the menstrual cycle.

• **Luteal phase:** When the egg leaves its follicle it travels down the Fallopian tube, brushed along by the cilia. The granulosa cells in the ruptured follicle form a structure called the corpus luteum. The release of LH from the pituitary gland immediately before ovulation stimulates the corpus luteum to produce a hormone called progesterone, which prepares the uterus for implantation of a developing embryo. If fertilisation does not happen and there is no embryo to implant, the corpus luteum breaks down and progesterone production falls. This causes the uterus to shed its lining resulting in a period (menstruation). This second half of the cycle is called the luteal phase and lasts 12 to 16 days. However, if a pregnancy does occur, the embryo produces a hormone called human chorionic gonadotrophin (hCG), which stimulates the corpus luteum to continue progesterone production so that the uterine lining remains and menstruation does not occur.

What else happens during the menstrual cycle?

Many women are aware of the effects of oestrogen and progesterone within their own body. Towards the end of the follicular phase the high levels of oestrogen change the amount and consistency of cervical mucus from sparse and tacky to abundant and stretchy, rather like egg white. This type of mucus allows sperm to enter and survive in the cervix.

The change from oestrogen to mainly progesterone after ovulation increases basal body temperature by 0.5 to 1.6°C, which may be used as a way of detecting that ovulation has occurred. Some women are aware of ovulation pains due to the inflammatory process, as the follicle gets ready to burst. These generally occur several hours before the actual time of rupture. Most women are also aware of premenstrual symptoms caused by the falling levels of both oestrogen and progesterone, which indicate that a period is about to begin.

Changes in the menstrual cycle with age

By the time a woman reaches her late thirties the number of eggs left in her ovaries will have fallen to around 20,000, and by her mid-forties there are only a few hundred left. The quality of the remaining eggs also declines with age, perhaps because healthier eggs are more likely to develop earlier, and perhaps because over the decades the eggs that were laid down before birth accumulate damage due to ageing. This is why by her later thirties a woman's chance per month of becoming pregnant falls dramatically and the incidence of miscarriage and chromosomal abnormality increases.

By her late forties, there are so few follicles at the right stage of development that some months will go by without any follicles reaching full development. Menstrual cycles become irregular and there are long periods when oestrogen is low and FSH is high. This is called the peri-menopause, which may last from a few months to a few years. The low levels of oestrogen are associated with hot flushes, mood changes and loss of bone density.

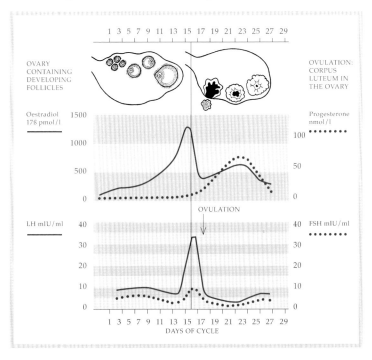

Figure 3: Schematic diagram of follicle growth in the ovary during the menstrual cycle.

Male reproductive system

In the male fetus, the migrating sex cells also end up in the tissue overlying the kidneys, which develop into the testes. Male sex hormones from the early testes cause the male reproductive system to develop. After this brief period of activity, the testes remain dormant until puberty.

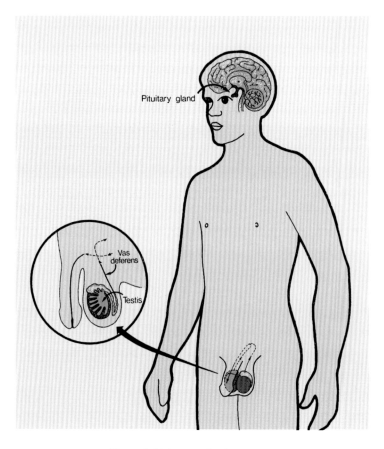

Figure 4: Male reproductive system.

Around puberty, the testes grow; the sex cells (spermatogonia) start to multiply and their progeny turn into sperm. Sperm production (spermatogenesis) depends on LH acting on the testes to make the hormone testosterone, and on FSH acting on specific stages of the maturing sperm. Testosterone is also responsible for male characteristics like body hair, a deep voice, muscle mass and some male behaviour.

Sperm production occurs within hundreds of long tubules that pack the testes. The end of each tubule empties into the epididymis, a gland sitting on the surface of the testis (see Figure 5). During passage through the epididymis, sperm undergo final maturation and acquire the ability to move. With ejaculation (orgasm) the sperm are transported rapidly along a tube called the vas deferens, past the seminal vesicles and prostate gland, which add seminal fluid, and out through the urethra, which runs through the penis. Any blockage in the system may result in a man being infertile.

The adult human testes make about a hundred million sperm a day. Despite their vast number, the sperm and fluid from the testes make up less than 5% of the volume of the ejaculate.

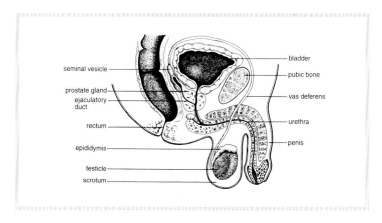

Figure 5: Male reproductive organs.

Fertilisation and conception

At ovulation, the egg literally bursts from its follicle and is taken up by the open end of the adjacent Fallopian tube. Although the egg is only about one-tenth of a millimetre across, it is embedded in a fluffy mass of granulosa cells which give the egg mass, with a diameter of 1–5 mm. From ovulation the egg has a 'use by' date of only 18–24 hours. Fortunately, sperm have longer lives, and can reliably survive in cervical mucus and in the Fallopian tube for two to three days.

Of the 200 million or so sperm ejaculated, only about 200 survive the journey and actually end up in the vicinity of the egg at the end of the Fallopian tube. Of those 200, only one sperm actually fertilises the egg.

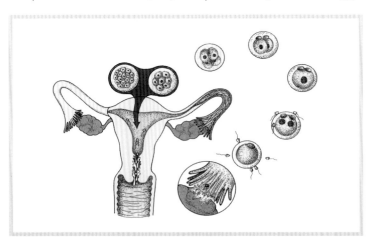

Figure 6: Schematic diagram showing the ovulated egg being picked up by the Fallopian tube and the stages of the embryo as it travels down the tube to the uterus.

Conception is not so much a moment as a process, during which egg meets sperm and fertilisation happens. This process, which lasts about 24 hours, begins with surface changes on the head of the sperm, giving it the capacity to fertilise an egg. Next the sperm loses part of its membrane, releasing enzymes into its immediate environment, which allow the sperm to make its way through the mass of granulosa cells attached to the egg. The sperm binds to the tough but flexible 'shell' of the egg (called the zona pellucida) and then dissolves its way through the zona by way of enzymes and whiplash movements. Once the successful sperm reaches the surface of the egg cell beneath the zona, it sets off electrical and chemical reactions within the egg to stop any further sperm from penetrating the egg. Eight to 12 hours later the egg has engulfed the sperm and the genetic material from the sperm and egg become organised into two pronuclei. These are clearly visible under a microscope and are proof of fertilisation. After another 12 hours, the two sets of genetic material merge; fertilisation is complete and the egg and the sperm have been transformed into an embryo.

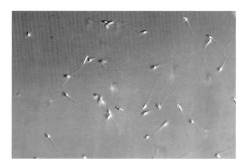

Figure 7: Sperm.

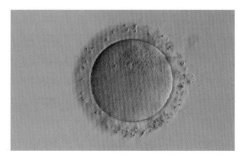

Figure 8: An egg surrounded by sperm.

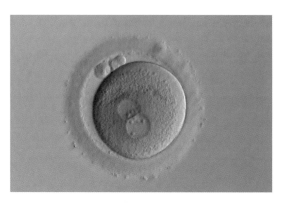

Figure 9: Fertilised egg. After fertilisation two pronuclei may be seen.

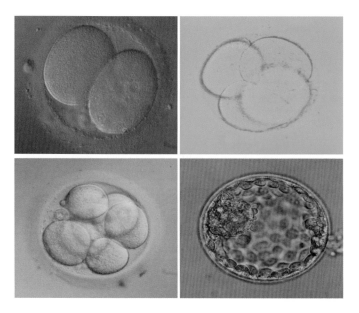

Figure 10: Top left and right: a 2-cell embryo (early day 2), a 4-cell embryo (late day 2). Bottom left and right: an 8-cell embryo (day 3), and a blastocyst (day 5).

The early embryo

The embryo begins cell division 28–34 hours after fertilisation and by 36–44 hours the embryonic cells have multiplied from one cell to four cells (see Figure 10).

If all goes well, the number of cells continues to increase to over 100, and by the fifth day the embryo has increased in complexity but not size, as it is still encased within its protective zona. During this time the embryo has been transported down the Fallopian tube into the uterus. At this stage the embryo is known as a blastocyst, a fragile fluid-filled ball, containing a mass of cells at one end, which develop into the fetus. On the fifth or sixth day, enzymes made by the embryo start to weaken the zona, which stretches and splits, allowing the embryo to 'hatch' and burrow into the uterine lining, where it begins to grow. This is known as implantation and is when the placenta starts to form.

Once out of the zona, the embryo needs an ever-increasing supply of nutrients and oxygen to support its enormous growth, which is supplied by the placenta. By the fifth week after the last menstrual period, a fetal sac filled with amniotic fluid can be seen in the uterus using ultrasound, and by the sixth week, a fetal heart can be detected.

How do twins form?

When two eggs are fertilised at the same time and implant together, non-identical twins develop. Identical twins arise from a single embryo that separates into two.

CHAPTER THREE

WHAT IS INFERTILITY?

This chapter examines human fertility and problems associated with infertility. Also, the disturbances that can cause a problem with conception are explored and some answers provided.

When is there a problem?

Having decided that you want to get pregnant, you stop contraception and go ahead and try. However, if as time passes you do not become pregnant, you may begin to wonder, worry and ask questions. One of those questions you may raise is: 'Is there a problem?'

Infertility is a silent problem. Usually there are no symptoms and it causes no overt disability. It has been defined as the failure to conceive after one year of unprotected intercourse, yet in reality infertility starts when a couple begins to fear that something may be wrong — often long before a year has passed. It is also defined by having more than two consecutive miscarriages or stillbirths. Infertility is a unique medical problem in that the 'patient' is a couple, both a man and a woman. Although historically always attributed to the woman, the cause lies nearly as often with the man.

Although infertility may be caused by a physical disease, such as tubal damage or impaired sperm production, the 'disease' of infertility is not usually experienced as an illness of the body but as a longing of the heart. Feelings of anger, denial, guilt, sadness, isolation, frustration and remorse are universal. Infertility also causes stress (although there is little evidence that stress causes infertility). But there is hope; most couples with 'infertility' will conceive eventually, with or without medical help.

Human fertility and the chances of pregnancy

At the best of times and, for some, no doubt the worst of times, getting pregnant is a matter of chance. There is even a definition for this chance; fecundability, which means the monthly probability of conception. The term fecundity is more often used, meaning the probability of a live birth resulting from one cycle of ovulation. Many people are surprised to hear that the human has a very low fecundity when compared to most other species. While this is not a problem for humans as a species, at a personal level it can give rise to great heartache. Although most of us know some couples that seem to conceive just by looking at each other, the average chance of conception from each ovulation is only 20 to 25%. This means that some couples with normal 'fertility' may take up to 18 months to achieve a pregnancy. As with all statistics in biology, findings there is a wide normal distribution range within the population. Taking this into account, fecundity in the human probably ranges from 0 to 60%. Zero fecundity means sterility.

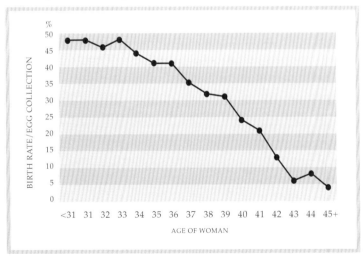

Figure 11a: Chance of pregnancy by age in an IVF programme.

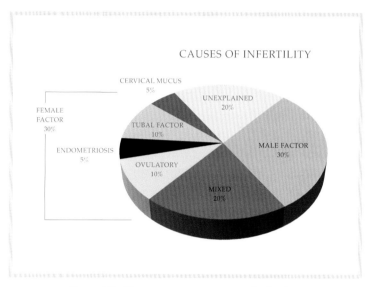

Figure 11b: The most common causes of infertility.

Bad eggs and bad sperm

If we consider the average couple with a 20 to 25% chance of conception, only 65% of those couples will have conceived within six months, which is usually when most couples start to feel concerned.

Sperm production and egg maturation are defective in the human compared to most mammals. Probably 30 to 40% of human eggs have an abnormal number or arrangement of chromosomes, which contain DNA (the genetic material in the cells). Although these defective eggs can be fertilised, embryo development nearly always stops soon after fertilisation. This is the major reason why even fertile couples have only a 20 to 25% chance of conceiving in any menstrual cycle, compared to 60 to 80% for cattle and sheep.

If humans were seasonal breeders like cattle or sheep this would present a terrible problem for the species, but since women can become pregnant throughout the year and have an extended reproductive span (20 to 25 years), compared to other species, this relative inefficiency is of little consequence. However, it is a problem when it comes to the treatment of infertility, because even if treatment (with IVF, for example) gives a normal chance of pregnancy, the highest success rate one can expect is still only 40 to 50% per month of treatment. The reason that IVF offers a higher chance of pregnancy compared with a natural cycle is because the best embryo can be chosen. In a natural cycle, there is no choice as usually only one egg is produced at ovulation.

In addition, the majority of sperm in the ejaculate of fertile men are deformed or dead, and the number of sperm produced per gram of testicular tissue is only one-quarter that of most mammals. However, so many sperm are ejaculated at once that enough sperm reach and surround the egg to ensure fertilisation.

Whatever happened to natural fertility?

With the advent of assisted reproductive technology, such as IVF, increased publicity about infertility would have us believe that this is a growing problem. However, figures are hard to come by because it is difficult to measure fertility in the general population.

There has been a well-documented increase in the incidence of sexually transmitted diseases which will, if not treated promptly, cause tubal damage resulting in infertility. Much concern has been voiced about a slow decline in sperm numbers in the average male ejaculate, and environmental toxins are often quoted as the cause. As yet there is little evidence to suggest that this decline is having an impact on human fertility.

Probably of much greater importance is the current trend of delaying having children until the woman is older and more secure. While this may be seen as of benefit to modern society, because it allows women to have a better education, travel and have a career, it also means that there is less time to fit in having children before fertility naturally declines with age.

The general consensus is that there has not been a great increase in the incidence of infertility but rather that more couples are seeking help, as treatments have become more accessible and effective.

What could be wrong?
Unexplained infertility
Knowledge of the basic physiology of conception (as explained in Chapter 2) will help you understand why it may take you a long time to conceive or indeed why it may not be possible for you to become pregnant. Understanding the complexity of the process may help explain why sometimes a reason is not found for a couple being unable to conceive. This is called 'unexplained infertility' and sometimes mistakenly suggests there is nothing wrong. However, there certainly is a problem, even though it may not be possible to define it. Unexplained infertility is usually the most frustrating type to deal with but the good news is that often, with time, couples will eventually conceive on their own, but if not, modern fertility treatments mean that help is available.

Sterility
Most couples equate infertility with sterility, which is not surprising as this is the usual dictionary definition, and this misunderstanding causes much anxiety. However, sterility means that a woman will never be able to conceive or a male induce conception, whereas infertility means a reduced or lost ability but does not automatically mean you will never be able to get pregnant. Only 5% of couples have problems of sterility (complete infertility), so for most couples the problem is of relative infertility or subfertility, meaning that they will usually conceive with time.

Factors that cause sterility are straightforward and easy to diagnose:
- azoospermia — no sperm
- anovulation — no ovulation
- menopause — no eggs

- blocked Fallopian tubes
- absent uterus

Unfortunately, if there is no treatment available, the couple will never be able to achieve a pregnancy.

Subfertility

Subfertility means that pregnancy is possible but the chances have been reduced due to a variety of possible reasons. From studies in Western countries it would appear that 20 to 25% of all couples who attempt to conceive experience an episode of subfertility at some stage of their reproductive lives.

About one in eight women experience this when attempting to conceive their first child (primary infertility) and one in six when attempting to conceive their second child (secondary infertility). Most couples will conceive with either time or treatment and so will have 'resolved' subfertility. Women who never conceive either with or without treatment have 'unresolved' infertility and various studies show that this occurs in 3 to 7% of couples who have never been able to become pregnant or who wanted more children but could not have them.

What causes infertility?

Unfortunately, factors that cause subfertility are more difficult to diagnose and the results of investigations are often inconclusive. The man is responsible in probably 30% of cases and contributory in another 20% of cases (see Figure 11b).

- **Problems with sperm:** Sperm are produced in the testes in enormous numbers and most men are impressed to hear that their sperm count is in the millions, although only hundreds reach the egg because there is a huge attrition between where sperm are deposited in the vagina and where they meet the egg.

Decreased numbers or motility of sperm reduces the chances of sperm reaching and fertilising the egg, which reduces the chance of a pregnancy. Although it is often quoted that 'it takes only one sperm', this is not true of natural conception since the process of fertilisation of the egg is a team event requiring hundreds of sperm. Following ejaculation, semen will coagulate for up to 30 minutes, allowing the sperm to swim into the cervical mucus.

When the semen liquefies, the fluid is lost via the vagina, an observation that may cause concern as the reason you are not getting pregnant, but this is not so.

• **Cervical mucus:** Changes in cervical mucus at ovulation is important in allowing sperm to get through the cervix and survive in the cervix for up to several days. Disorders of the mucus, which usually result from operations to the cervix such as laser treatment, can interfere with this process.

• **Uterine problems:** Uterine problems causing infertility are rare but may interfere with the transport of sperm through the uterus, which is thought to involve uterine contractions and may also interfere with implantation. These problems include fibroids, polyps, adhesions and congenital abnormalities.

• **Tubal problems:** Blocked tubes are a common cause of infertility. Delicate finger-like processes, or fimbria, at the ends of each tube collect the egg and help to guide it into the Fallopian tube. Blockage or scarring of the fimbria will interfere with conception. The cilia lining the tube can also be damaged by infection and, as they are very important for embryo transport, this can also interfere with conception.

• **Ovulation problems:** Disruption or lack of ovulation will also decrease or abolish any chances of conception and about 10% of infertility is due to problems with ovulation. These may be due to a hormonal imbalance.

A common cause of irregular ovulation is a condition known as polycystic ovarian syndrome (PCOS), in which ovarian follicles stop growing past a certain size. The ovary accumulates lots of medium-sized fluid-filled, non-functional follicles. These cystic follicles produce more androgen than usual, giving rise to the common symptoms of acne and excessive hair growth.

Other symptoms are less obvious; women with polycystic ovaries have an increased risk of developing diabetes and often have an abnormal response to insulin.

• **Endometriosis:** This condition is described in Chapter 4 and is where implants of endometrium in the pelvis cause an inflammatory process which may cause infertility. Common symptoms associated with endometriosis include severe period pain, spotting pre-period and pain during sex.

• **Combination of factors:** While infertility may be caused by one well-defined factor, it can also be the result of a combination of lesser factors, which, if present in isolation, may cause no problem but when put together will cause profound infertility.

Probably the most common combination of problems is a decreased sperm count and endometriosis. Endometriosis is discussed in more detail in Chapter 4, later in the book.

When to seek help?

There is no right answer, but if you are concerned, then perhaps this is a good time to seek help. Most couples who conceive spontaneously will do so in the first six months, so if within six months you are not pregnant and worried that there may be a problem, it is reasonable to see a doctor at this point. There are circumstances when earlier advice should be sought, such as:

- lack of regular periods
- known low sperm count
- a previous operation to bring down a testis into the scrotum as a child
- previous treatments for cancer in either partner

When to investigate infertility will depend very much on a couple's wishes, but generally it is best to begin investigations as soon as you have concerns that there may be a problem. Since infertility is a problem for you both as a couple it is important that both partners be tested.

In some cases you may be encouraged to wait a while before any invasive tests are performed, for example, if you have been trying for only a few months, the woman is under 35, and there is nothing to suggest an anatomical problem.

Paradoxically, couples who may need longer to conceive because the woman is older, require earlier investigations because there is less time left for conception. If the likelihood that there is a problem is greater — for example, because of a history of male infertility in the family, undescended testes, irregular periods or previous pelvic infection — then prompt investigations may be indicated, sometimes even before you start trying to conceive.

Diagnostic testing will reveal only the most obvious and severe abnormalities. Sometimes no cause will be found, which everyone finds very frustrating.

Chapters 5 and 6 explain what is involved in investigation into infertility in men and women.

CHAPTER FOUR

ENDOMETRIOSIS

Endometriosis is a condition that affects many women of reproductive age, as many as 10 to 15% of New Zealand women, probably more, as it is not always recognised.

For many women endometriosis may have a major impact on their lives, causing pain or infertility, so appropriate and expert medical care is essential. This chapter explains how endometriosis can be involved in infertility and what can be done for women with this condition to improve the chances of becoming pregnant.

What is endometriosis?

The endometrium is the tissue that normally lines the uterus. Endometriosis occurs when endometrial tissue grows outside the uterus and causes a chronic inflammatory reaction. This tissue may implant anywhere in the pelvis or abdomen, including the Fallopian tubes and ovaries or, more rarely, may be found in distant sites such as skin or lungs. The tissue may grow in small patches or may infiltrate deeply into other surrounding tissues, or may form cysts in the ovaries.

Endometriosis is notoriously unpredictable. Some women have a few isolated spots (see Figure 12), which may regress, whilst others have a progressive form of the disease, which spreads throughout the entire pelvis (see Figure 13).

Because endometrial tissue behaves in the same way wherever it is, responding to the female hormones oestrogen and progesterone, and preparing the uterus for a possible pregnancy by thickening and increasing the blood supply, this can cause a lot of pain, discomfort and heavy menstrual bleeding. Endometriosis also irritates the surrounding tissue, which can result in the formation of scar tissue (adhesions), and these adhesions may cause pelvic organs, like the uterus and the bowel, to bind to one another.

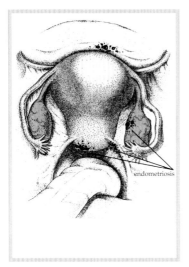

Figure 12: Pelvis showing mild endometriosis. The lines indicate black areas of endometriosis.

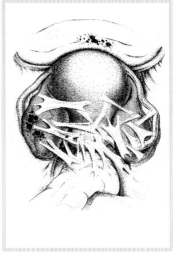

Figure 13: Severe endometriosis with thick scar tissue and adhesions.

What causes endometriosis?

We don't know what causes endometriosis. The most popular theory is retrograde menstruation, which is where menstrual blood flows along the Fallopian tubes and is deposited in the pelvis, whereupon some of the endometrial cells implant, causing endometriosis. However, all women have some menstrual blood deposited in their pelvis each month and yet not all women develop endometriosis. It is likely that there is a genetic predisposition for endometriosis and that inherited genes may confer a higher risk of endometriosis. If you have a mother or sister with endometriosis you are nine times more likely to also have the disease. Other possibilities for the cause of endometriosis include involvement of the immune system and environmental toxins such as dioxins. Further work is being done in this area.

Can endometriosis cause infertility?

The relationship between endometriosis and infertility is not completely understood, although between 20 and 40% of women with infertility will have endometriosis. Endometriosis may cause infertility by causing adhesions. Another possibility is that the production of chemical messengers called cytokines produced as a result of the inflammation may interfere with the process of sperm meeting egg or they may alter tubal transport.

Endometriosis is more commonly diagnosed in women who are being investigated for infertility as compared to women who are having a laparoscopy for sterilisation. Women who are known to have endometriosis usually take longer to conceive than women without a prior diagnosis of the disease. However, many women with endometriosis do not have difficulty in conceiving. There is also no evidence that miscarriages occur more commonly in women with endometriosis.

Medical treatment for endometriosis (pills and injections) has not been found to improve fertility. Surgical treatment, in which the deposits of endometriosis are removed, does improve fertility. Sometimes IVF is needed, particularly with severe endometriosis.

What are the symptoms?

Some women experience severe symptoms and yet have only a few deposits of endometriosis, whilst others have severe disease with little or no symptoms. The most common symptoms experienced by women with endometriosis include:

- painful periods, which are the most common symptom and while many women have pain with their periods, pain associated with endometriosis may start some days before bleeding and tends to be more severe
- period pain that gets progressively more severe with age
- pain during sex (dyspareunia), which may be caused by deposits of endometriosis at the top of the vagina or on the ligaments behind the uterus which are stretched during sex

- chronic fatigue
- bloating
- bowel problems, such as pain when going to the toilet, or constipation
- bleeding irregularities, such as premenstrual spotting
- occasional bladder symptoms linked with periods
- infertility

How is endometriosis diagnosed

Doctors are notoriously slow at diagnosing endometriosis and the average duration of symptoms is nine years before a diagnosis is made. Endometriosis cannot be diagnosed on symptoms alone, but requires direct observation using laparoscopy or another surgical procedure.

Appearance under laparoscopy

Endometriosis has many different appearances in the pelvis. It may look like small flecks of paint on the pelvic surfaces. Often thick scar tissue is the only finding, with adhesions that may bind the uterus, tubes, ovaries or bowel together. Ovarian cysts caused by endometriosis tend to be filled with blood and with time this blood becomes dark brown in colour, which is why they are described as 'chocolate cysts'. These cysts may be as small as a pea or larger than a grapefruit. Occasionally the cysts may burst, leading to pain and the formation of more scar tissue.

Imaging

Various imaging technologies, such as ultrasound, magnetic resonance imaging (MRI) or computerised tomography (CT) may be used to diagnose the extent of the endometriosis.

What is the treatment?

Surgical options

If you have picked up this book it means that fertility is your priority and this usually indicates surgery as the first treatment option. Surgery may

CASE HISTORY

Nira always had incredibly painful periods and usually needed to go home from school on the first two days of her period. Her family doctor told her that period pain was to be expected. At university she plucked up the courage to see a specialist who tried various pain-relieving options without success. Eventually, Nira had a laparoscopy, which revealed very extensive endometriosis in her pelvis. The endometriosis was removed and Nira was put on the pill. Nira's symptoms were better but she still needed painkillers to get through the first two days of her period. After one year of infertility Nira saw a fertility specialist who advised a repeat laparoscopy. This procedure showed severe disease. An endometriotic cyst was removed from the ovary and the specialist recommended IVF treatment. Nira and her partner conceived on their first cycle of IVF using a frozen embryo.

be used to remove chocolate cysts and implants of endometriosis, to divide adhesions and to restore normal anatomy. Laparoscopic surgery is advancing all the time, so most women with endometriosis may be treated with minimal external scars and short hospital stays. Most women have significant relief of pain following surgical removal of endometriosis. If you have endometriosis, surgery will improve your chances of conception.

Pregnancy

Pregnancy is sometimes said to be the best treatment for endometriosis, as the condition tends to regress during pregnancy. However, this may be impossible to achieve, or it may not be appropriate for some women at that time in their lives. Endometriosis usually causes no problems during pregnancy and most women find their endometriosis symptoms go away after the birth, but in time symptoms can return.

Hormonal medication

Hormonal medication is useful for the relief of pain but is not curative and does not improve the chances of pregnancy. The rationale behind hormonal therapy in endometriosis is to mimic the menopause

> ## CASE HISTORY
> Claire, a 36-year-old lawyer, is married to Neil, a property developer. Claire had always had severe period pain and, since coming off the pill eight months ago, this became much worse. A laparoscopy was performed, which revealed normal tubes but moderate endometriosis, which was excised. Claire's periods improved over the next few months and six months after surgery she became pregnant.

or pregnancy as both of these conditions cause a regression in endometriosis. Hormonal therapy suppresses ovarian activity and prevents both the normal endometrium and the extra endometrial tissue from being stimulated to grow each month. Whilst on hormonal medications for endometriosis you will not be able to become pregnant because of the adverse hormonal environment.

Hormonal treatments used include:
- the oral contraceptive pill taken continuously
- danazol or gestrinone
- progestogens
- gonadotrophin-releasing hormone analogues
- the Mirena intrauterine contraceptive device

All of these medications have side effects and women should discuss their relative benefits and risks with a clinician who has experience in this field. There is no evidence that hormonal medication improves fertility in women with endometriosis once they stop medication, but many women do have significant relief from painful symptoms. However, these symptoms may return once the medication is stopped. Large chocolate ovarian cysts do not respond to hormonal treatments and surgery is often required.

Lifestyle advice
Living with chronic pain can be very difficult. The New Zealand Endometriosis Foundation is a useful support group. It advises you take regular exercise, and increase fruit, vegetables, nuts and seeds in your diet. Some women find certain foods, such as dairy, coffee and high-fat diets, may aggravate the symptoms.

PAINKILLERS
Paracetamol
Codeine
Non-steroidal anti-inflammatory drugs, eg, Ponstan or Synflex
HORMONAL TREATMENTS
Oral contraceptive pill taken continuously
Progestogens, eg, Provera
Danazol
Gestrinone
Gonadatrophin-releasing hormone analogues
The Mirena intrauterine device
SURGICAL TREATMENTS
Laparoscopic removal of endometriosis using diathermy, laser or excision
Laparotomy
Hysterectomy

Table 2: Management of endometriosis.

Fertility treatment in women with endometriosis

If you have mild endometriosis and no other cause for infertility, it is wise to allow extra time to see if you can become pregnant spontaneously. For older women (37 or more), or for couples who have been unable to conceive for two or more years, it is worthwhile considering some form of assisted conception. Either intrauterine insemination (IUI), with ovarian stimulation, or IVF would be suitable treatments. Women with endometriosis have the same chances of conception using IVF as couples with other causes for their infertility. If the problem is extensive ovarian endometriosis, then you may produce fewer eggs in an IVF cycle and may need a stronger ovarian stimulation regime. Once pregnant, endometriosis does not tend to cause problems.

If you have endometriosis and your partner has suboptimal sperm, often IVF is needed as the presence of two fertility problems make spontaneous conception much less likely to occur.

After pregnancy and breastfeeding, endometriosis may be suppressed for some time allowing an opportunity for conception to occur.

CHAPTER FIVE

TESTS AND INVESTIGATIONS FOR FEMALE INFERTILITY

It is commonly said that because a woman's reproductive system is more complicated than a man's she has to undergo more invasive tests to discover the reason why she cannot become pregnant.

Unfortunately, this is partly true because tubal investigations are more complex and do carry a risk. Investigations are designed to answer some basic questions about a woman's fertility:

- is ovulation normal?
- is the cervical mucus normal?
- are the uterus and tubes normal?

Is ovulation happening?

Normal cycle

Almost all women who do not ovulate will have an irregular or absent menstrual cycle. Regular cycles are linked with easily identified monthly changes, like premenstrual symptoms of bloating and breast discomfort, cramping pain with the first day of bleeding, and changes in mid-cycle mucus. Women who experience these changes will be ovulating. It is unusual for a normal cycle length to be exactly the average 28-day cycle every month (unless on the pill). Normal cycles ranging from 21 to 35 days are common and are usually ovulatory. It is also normal for a cycle to vary by two to three days each month.

Basal body temperature

When ovulation happens your basal body temperature increases by 0.5 to 1.6°C, which can be picked up if you keep regular temperature charts. We mention this only because it is still commonly described as a method of detecting ovulation. Although simple and inexpensive, it is stressful for most couples because it interferes with the spontaneity of sex and can be a constant reminder of your problem. 'There are three of us in bed — me, my partner and the thermometer' is a common feeling. Also, ovulation can only be detected in hindsight, making this a method to be discouraged.

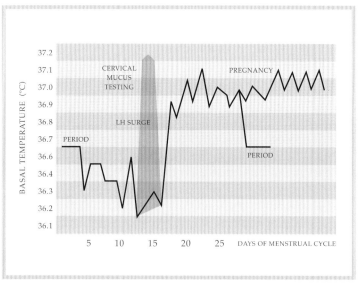

Figure 14: Basal body temperature chart.

Mucus changes

Cervical mucus changes in consistency at the time of ovulation (as described in Chapter 1) and these changes follow a characteristic pattern of a dry vaginal sensation followed by a wet sensation, then a dry sensation, ending with a period 14 days later. This pattern is good evidence that ovulation is occurring and also, unlike the basal body temperature chart, can be used to ensure you have intercourse as close to ovulation day as possible, enhancing your chances of conceiving.

Blood tests for hormone levels

Having the right amount of the right hormones in your blood at the right time of the monthly cycle is critical for ovulation to happen. We discussed the various female hormones and their roles in the menstrual cycle in Chapter 2. Here we explain the blood tests to measure levels of these hormones that will help find out if all is well.

• **Follicle stimulating hormone (FSH):** FSH is measured on day two of the menstrual cycle, to estimate whether you have a reasonable number of eggs remaining in your ovaries. A normal FSH level is between one and 10 IU/Litre, and these levels increase as menopause approaches reflecting the lack of eggs. The FSH level is also used to determine the dose of drugs to be used in an IVF cycle. Measuring FSH is not a perfect test and newer tests are being developed which may predict the ovarian reserve with more accuracy. An oestradiol level (oestradiol is a form of oestrogen) is measured at the same time, as an FSH level may only be interpreted in conjunction with an oestradiol level.

• **Progesterone:** Appropriately timed blood tests for progesterone are usually the only confirmation of ovulation needed if you have a history of regular menstrual cycles, as it is produced after ovulation by the egg follicle once it has released the egg (corpus luteum). Appropriate timing means a blood test six to eight days after ovulation and not day 21 of the menstrual cycle as commonly requested.

• **Luteinising hormone (LH):** If it is necessary to know the exact day of ovulation then daily testing for LH will provide you with this information, as LH levels increase at the time of ovulation. You can measure LH in your urine using a self-testing kit and this can be done at home. Although blood levels of LH give a more accurate assessment of the time of ovulation, it is not often done except for a post-coital test or treatments such as intrauterine insemination.

• **Anti-Müllerian hormone (AMH):** Anti-Müllerian hormone is made by small follicles in the ovaries. It can be measured in a blood test at any time in the menstrual cycle, or even in women on the oral contraceptive pill. AMH can pick up who might lose their fertility more quickly.

Investigating structural problems

Anatomical problems of the uterus, tubes and ovaries can seldom be predicted from a woman's medical history. Also, they usually do not give rise to any symptoms and are not usually detectable on examination. There are several tests that can be carried out to investigate whether there are any structural problems. Some of these investigations are invasive, particularly tests for pelvic assessment, and do require a hospital visit. These include hysterosalpingogram, which better assesses the lumen of the tubes, whereas a laparoscopy is a much more accurate investigation and allows the pelvic organs to be visualised and any operative manoeuvres performed.

Ultrasound

A pelvic ultrasound is usually performed at the first visit to determine if everything is in good working order and whether there are any structural problems. Ultrasound can pick up:

• **Uterine problems:** The size and shape of the uterus is investigated, as well as checking for fibroids or polyps. Occasionally other radiological techniques may be used as part of fertility investigations, such as an MRI of the uterus if fibroids are diagnosed on ultrasound. Sometimes saline is infused through the cervix and an ultrasound scan is used to determine whether the uterine cavity is normal (saline sonogram).

• **Ovarian health:** Ovaries are also examined, as ultrasound can detect ovarian cysts along with providing an indication of ovarian reserve by measuring the tiny follicles present in the ovaries, which will mature and produce eggs (antral follicle count). It is possible to see the growth of the follicle in the ovary (see Figure 15); a follicle can ovulate when its average size is between 16–30 mm and it grows at a rate of 2–3 mm a day. The condition of polycystic ovaries can be diagnosed using ultrasound.

• **Ovulation timing:** Ultrasound is not used to predict the exact time of ovulation. It is used to detect the development of more than one follicle when stimulatory drugs are used and to enable accurate timing of the

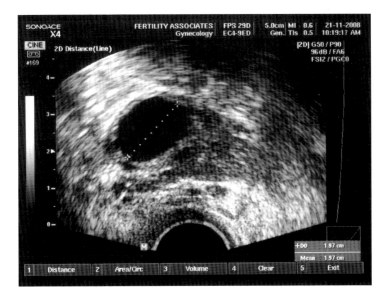

Figure 15: Ultrasound showing an ovary with a dark area
which is the developing follicle.

triggering of ovulation when the largest follicle is of adequate size.

• **Fallopian tubes:** An ultrasound does not detect tubal problems unless large blocked tubes are present (hydrosalpinges).

Hysterosalpingogram

This is an X-ray of the uterus and tubes and is often referred to as an HSG (see Figure 16). This procedure does not require a general anaesthetic, although it can give rise to some discomfort. A dye, which shows up on X-ray, is introduced through the cervix and passes through the uterus and tubes, so that when an X-ray is taken an outline of both the uterine cavity and the inside of the tubes is shown. The X-ray will show whether there is a blockage in the tubes and also where the blockage is.

Unfortunately, the test sometimes gives false results, so it is not foolproof but is best used to complement other tests, such as laparoscopic findings of tubal disease; it also helps to define

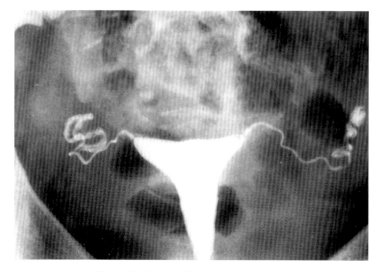

Figure 16: A normal hysterosalpingogram.

more clearly the inside, in particular the inner end, of the Fallopian tube. An HSG can also help assess the uterine cavity and identify problems with the uterus, although hysteroscopy is usually used for investigations of the uterus.

Hysteroscopy and laparoscopy

These procedures are usually performed at the same time under a general anaesthetic. A telescope called a hysteroscope is introduced through the cervix into the uterus, giving an excellent view of the uterine cavity. Another telescope called a laparoscope is introduced into the abdomen through a small incision in the tummy button, to view the pelvic organs and fully assess the peritoneal surfaces (lining of the abdominal cavity) covering the uterus, tubes and ovaries so that any adhesions or endometriosis may be found (see Figure 17). The patency of the tubes is checked by injecting dye through the cervix and watching its passage through the outer ends of the tubes. The assessment is

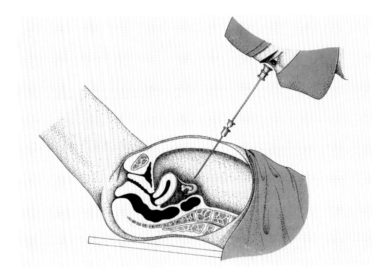

Figure 17: Diagram of a laparoscopy.

dependent on the experience and skill of the operator and is best done by a fertility surgeon. If problems are found, then surgery can be performed at the same time. These procedures are done on an outpatient basis and you can usually go home a few hours after the procedure, although you will need a further three to four days off work.

What next?

The introduction of successful treatments for infertility that do not depend on knowing the exact cause of the problem has meant that the need for these investigations has been revised. If they are inconclusive, rather than pursuing more intense investigations it is best to allocate some time to try for pregnancy or consider treatment. This will depend on the length of infertility and the time left for conception. The latter is usually defined by the age of the woman. These factors, rather than the cause of the infertility, will usually define when a couple should progress to treatment.

CHAPTER SIX

MALE INFERTILITY EXPLORED

One of the most devastating things a man can be told is that his sperm test is abnormal. This chapter discusses the causes, likely investigations, options and lifestyle measures available to men when there is a sperm issue.

Sperm problems are very common and 40% of couples having difficulties conceiving are found to have a lower quality semen analysis. Often there is a mild problem in both partners, which can contribute to a couple's inability to conceive, and it is only when they occur together that they result in infertility. The trend for increased age in couples starting a family means that this delay in attempting to conceive may add to any male problem, as an older woman is less able to compensate as her own fertility has declined.

There is a distinct possibility that sperm problems are increasing in frequency, possibly due to chemicals in the environment which may disrupt the normal development of the testes. There are many other reasons for sperm problems and there are things you can do to improve sperm quality.

Sperm problems may be broadly put into two major categories, genetic or environmental causes, and both are discussed in this chapter.

Genetic causes of sperm problems

Genetic causes tend to result in very severe abnormalities. Up to 15% of men with zero or very low sperm counts have small pieces of the Y chromosome missing (micro-deletions) and this, along with the sperm problems it causes, will be inherited by boys conceived from fathers with this micro-deletion.

Other genetic causes include cystic fibrosis, which is an inherited disease. This prevents normal formation of the ducts from the testes so that sperm cannot be released from the testes and then be ejaculated. If other men in your family have fertility issues then you are more likely to also have fertility issues as it is thought that there is an inherited predisposition for fertility.

Environmental causes of sperm problems

Environmental causes of sperm problems may happen during fetal life, childhood or even in adult life. Here are some examples, although in most cases no cause can be found, which is very frustrating for all concerned.

Surgery or trauma

• If you had an operation as a child to bring down the testes into the scrotum, then there is a reasonable likelihood of also having a serious sperm problem. This operation is now performed on toddlers as the longer the testes remain in the warmer abdominal cavity, the more likely it is that sperm production may be affected as an adult.
• Any serious trauma to the testes, such as a rugby game injury, or testicular twisting or 'torsion', can affect sperm production.

Infection

• Mumps is often cited as a cause of male infertility, but it is rare and will only impair fertility if it occurs after puberty and causes the testes to become very swollen, always a memorable event in a man's life.
• Other infections such as gonorrhoea or chlamydia may cause blockage in the tubules.

Drugs and medication

• Chemotherapy can also impact on sperm production and this damage is often permanent as the sperm-producing cells are damaged.
• Occasionally other drugs may also compromise sperm, for example steroids used by bodybuilders, although often when drugs are stopped sperm production returns to normal.

CASE HISTORY

Julie and Chris were both keen triathletes. They looked after themselves well, exercised regularly, had a healthy diet and did not drink or smoke. Julie had very regular menstrual cycles so they were surprised they hadn't conceived after a year of trying. Julie was 34 and Chris had forgotten that when he was eight, he had an operation to bring his testes down. Their GP ordered a semen analysis which showed a very low sperm count. They were referred to a fertility clinic and are on the waiting list for IVF/ICSI treatment.

Chris has found the news very hard to take as he has always looked after his body and works in the health industry. To help their relationship cope they have decided to visit a counsellor.

Environmental toxins

There has been increasing interest recently in the effects of environmental toxins on male fertility. There appears to have been a steady decline in sperm counts over the last few decades, particularly in some countries in the industrialised world, including New Zealand. Environmental toxins are being looked at as a potential cause, and certain occupational groups who work amongst toxic fumes, insecticides, solvents, plastics, preservatives or lead are being monitored. Considerable research is also being done on the effect of phyto-oestrogens (oestrogens in plants) on sperm count, motility, structure and fertility. Although a definitive answer may be some time away there is a strong suspicion that environmental toxins are playing a substantial role in reduced fertility in some men.

Radiation

Radiation can kill the sperm-producing cells. Lower doses of radiation (and some toxic drugs) can damage sperm at particular stages of the maturation process, so that sperm can disappear from the ejaculate for several months or sometimes permanently.

Overheated testes

Men's testes are located outside the body cavity as heat is bad for sperm production. If the temperature of the testis is increased from its usual 33°C, for example by fever, sperm production can be greatly reduced for weeks. Permanently raising the temperature of the testes to 37°C has a profound effect on sperm survival.

It is thought that excessive heat may explain low sperm counts in men in wheelchairs, sedentary jobs or drivers such as taxi drivers or long-distance truckers. Some simple lifestyle measures may aid sperm production, such as wearing boxers instead of briefs and avoiding hot spas, saunas or baths.

In 2004, researchers at the State University of New York warned young men to limit the time they used their laptops on their laps, after tests showed that heat from the battery may impair sperm production. It is not known as yet whether keeping a mobile phone in your trouser pocket has any influence on sperm production.

What type of sperm problems are there?
No sperm

If there are no sperm present when you produce your first ejaculate sample, it should be repeated. If the same results are seen, the next step is to determine whether or not sperm are being produced by the testes. There are several explanations:

• If sperm are produced, but because of a plumbing problem in the tubing the sperm are not being ejaculated, they can almost always be retrieved from the testes by putting a small needle into the testes under local anaesthetic. Sperm retrieved directly from the testes can be frozen for use in an IVF cycle, but they need to be injected into eggs as they are not fully motile. In this scenario, the testes are normal sized and hormone levels are normal.

• Occasionally sperm are being produced by the testes but are being diverted into the bladder by valve problems, resulting in a very low volume of ejaculate. This can be caused by trauma or diabetes.

However, sperm can be obtained for insemination from the bladder.
• Some men have no sperm-producing cells in their testes which means that no sperm can be obtained. Others have occasional clusters of sperm-producing cells in their testes which can sometimes be found by performing a needle biopsy.

Sperm antibodies
Sperm antibodies coat the sperm, reducing their ability to swim normally through the female reproductive system, or block sperm recognition of the egg. This action therefore inhibits fertilisation and causes infertility. These antibodies are seen most commonly following a vasectomy reversal and can also appear following trauma to the testes or testicular surgery. It is only possible to test for sperm antibodies in a specialised fertility laboratory and, if found, the appropriate treatment is IVF with micro-injection of the sperm into the egg. If a post-coital test is performed with abnormal results, then a sperm antibody test is advised. Sperm antibody screening has become a routine test before IVF or IUI treatments.

Varicocele
A varicocele is a collection of varicose veins surrounding the testes. This is a common problem and varicoceles occur in about 40% of men having infertility problems. There is ongoing debate whether varicocele causes fertility issues; however, the consensus is that they may cause the testicular temperature to rise and thus affect sperm production. Varicocele may be treated by tying off the veins in a small operation or by an X-ray technique. There is, however, no evidence that treating a varicocele will improve sperm quality, probably because the operation should be done earlier in life.

Vasectomy
If you have previously had a vasectomy there is every chance that you will be able to have children, as a vasectomy can be reversed, which results in a successful pregnancy about half of the time. The

shorter the interval between the vasectomy and its reversal the greater chance of success. A vasectomy reversal is usually performed as day case surgery and follow-up sperm tests should be done to determine whether the operation has been successful. If your partner does not become pregnant, IVF with sperm micro-injection is a further option. If there are still no sperm in the ejaculate after a reversal operation then sperm may still be retrieved from the testes for use in an IVF cycle.

Semen analysis

A semen analysis is the most widely used test because it is so simple and it does provide important basic information. The most important aspect of a semen analysis is the number of motile (moving) sperm present.

Sample collection

• The semen is best collected by masturbation following two or three days' abstinence.

• The sample should be collected into a laboratory specimen container rather than using a normal condom as most condoms have spermicides which kill the sperm. If you wish to collect a sample using a condom, a fertility clinic can supply a silastic condom, which does not affect sperm.

• The semen should be kept at room temperature and taken to the laboratory for examination, ideally within one hour of collection.

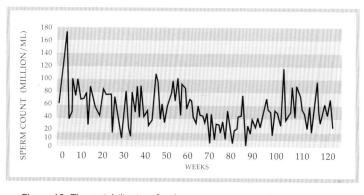

Figure 18: The variability in a fertile man's sperm count over two years.

Sperm assessment

An assessment of sperm in the semen sample you have provided involves several parameters. These are shown in the table below along with the normal values:

PARAMETER	NORMAL VALUE
Measuring the volume	Volume of 1–6 mls
Counting the sperm	• Greater than 20 million sperm/ml • Greater than 40 million sperm per ejaculate
Estimating the % of the sperm that are moving (motility)	• Greater than 40% progressive motility
Assessing the shape (morphology) and movement of the sperm	Sperm with normal structure and form: • Greater than 50% using conventional grading, or • Greater than 10% using 'strict' grading
Checking for sperm antibodies	None
Look for the presence of infection	None

However, sperm assessment does have limitations in that many men with results in the abnormal range are fertile but are just taking longer on average to produce a pregnancy. Some men with 'normal' results may have a major problem with sperm function. A fertility laboratory will be able to provide more useful results compared to the local community laboratory.

Variability in results

There can be wide variations in sperm count values just with time. Also, it is well known that severe infection can temporarily depress sperm counts for several months after an illness. If the semen analysis is abnormal it should be repeated over the ensuing months before conclusions are drawn (see Figure 18).

Blood tests for hormones

Blood tests for levels of follicle stimulating hormone (FSH), luteinising hormone (LH) and testosterone are performed when the sperm count is very low or absent. FSH is responsible for sperm production and if elevated can signal major sperm production problems. LH is responsible for triggering the production of testosterone by the testes. Prolactin is another hormone measured, particularly if impotence is an issue, as it is involved in libido and normal sex drive.

Other sperm tests

• **Chromosome analysis:** The chromosomes are also analysed if the sperm count is very low or there are no sperm present.

• **Sperm DNA fragmentation:** Newer tests have recently been developed, which can examine the integrity of the DNA in sperm. High levels of DNA damage may mean pregnancy is less likely and early pregnancy loss is more likely. It is not yet clear what intervention will improve DNA damage in sperm, but current suggestions include frequent ejaculation, antioxidant supplementation or possibly the use of sperm retrieved directly from the testes.

• **Post-coital test:** This test is not done very often but is a test for sperm function. Correct timing is essential and it must be performed a day before or on the day of ovulation. This can be monitored by detecting mid-cycle mucus changes or a self-test urinary kit for LH. A specimen of the mucus is examined microscopically within four to 18 hours after intercourse to look for sperm. If large numbers of motile sperm are visible, sperm function is likely to be good.

• **Ultrasound of testes:** An ultrasound examination of the testes is usually recommended whenever there is a significant abnormality following semen analysis or a physical examination. This may detect varicoceles (varicose veins around the testes), premalignant growths and cancers.

• **Biopsy of the testis:** A biopsy is only necessary in cases where no sperm have been found in the ejaculate following semen analysis and it is not clear from other tests whether or not sperm are being produced. It involves removing a small piece of testicular tissue under local anaesthetic for microscopic examination; if sperm are retrieved during the biopsy they are frozen for future use. The following table provides some lifestyle choices you can make that may improve sperm quality.

HOW TO KEEP SPERM HEALTHY AND IMPROVE SPERM QUALITY
Ensure your testes remain cool, as sperm production is markedly impaired by heat.
Don't smoke! Cigarette smoking damages the DNA in the sperm as well as increases the chances of your child developing childhood cancer fourfold.
Recreational drugs such as marijuana also adversely affect sperm.
Alcohol in large quantities reduces sperm production; the current recommendation is fewer than 20 units of alcohol per week.
Obesity also impacts on sperm production, with recent studies showing obese men having sperm counts 20% lower than men who are not obese.
A diet rich in antioxidants is likely to improve sperm quality. Eat foods such as brightly coloured fruit and vegetables like blueberries and tomatoes, along with nuts and seeds. Red wine, dark chocolate and green tea are also high in antioxidants.
Supplements containing vitamin C, E, selenium and zinc could possibly improve sperm. A new men's supplement 'Menevit' has recently been introduced to New Zealand and is available by prescription through fertility clinics. There has been one study showing that men who took 'Menevit' for three months prior to an IVF/ICSI (Intracytoplasmic Sperm Injection) cycle had better pregnancy rates compared to others who took a placebo pill.
Frequent ejaculation probably also improves sperm quality, as sperm can be damaged by free radicals while they are stored in the epididymis prior to ejaculation.

What next?

If hormonal abnormality is found, it is possible that medication may help in some cases, however, in most instances of male infertility there is no medication that will improve sperm quality. There are fortunately several treatment options available for assisted reproduction, as well as some natural and alternative therapies. These are discussed in the next chapter.

CHAPTER SEVEN

TREATMENT FOR INFERTILITY

Couples facing infertility now in the early 21st century have an enormous advantage over previous generations. For the first time in history there is reliable and safe technology that can give almost everyone a good chance of having a child.

We tend to forget how recent and momentous the changes have been. Even in the 1960s, the decade of the contraceptive pill, almost nothing could be done for infertility. While the first IVF child was born in 1977, it took another decade before IVF became widely available, and even then pregnancy rates were modest. It has only been in the last 10 years or so that pregnancy rates have significantly improved and that IVF technology has become helpful in resolving severe male infertility as well as female problems.

This chapter outlines the type of treatments available for 'assisted reproduction' and for whom they are useful. We start with 'lo-tech' options, including lifestyle and medical approaches, then discuss some 'mid-tech' options, including simple surgical procedures. Finally we move to 'hi-tech' options, including IVF and some newer, more advanced, technologies. There are also other options which we discuss, including the use of donors to provide sperm, eggs, embryos or even a surrogate uterus.

What is your game plan?

Many people have options about where to start treatment. Most choose to start with the simplest (and cheapest) option. Wherever you start, it is important to have a plan for what treatment you are willing to try, what to do next and how long you will give it a go before moving on to the next step. While many couples are lucky and become pregnant on their first or second treatment, it is your staying power and ability to persevere that gives you the best chance of having a child. For this reason we encourage people to look after their 'emotional stamina' as much as their physical health. We actively promote fertility counselling as a way of getting the information and skills you need to handle the emotional ups and downs of fertility treatment.

What your game plan should include

• **Age:** A crucial aspect of the 'game plan' is a woman's age; you can't turn back the clock but you can use what time you have wisely.

• **Action:** Don't delay; most couples who succeed in getting pregnant are those who get on with treatment without much delay.

• **Technology:** Decide what level of complexity you are comfortable with, in terms of technology available.

• **Counselling:** Consider counselling as part of your support plan for success.

A healthy body weight for ovulation

Many women who do not ovulate (sometimes called 'amenorrhea' meaning no menstrual periods) or who have irregular ovulation ('oligomenorrhea' meaning few menstrual periods) are over or under the ideal body weight for their height. Women whose body mass index (BMI) is below 19 are encouraged to gain weight and those with a BMI above 27 are strongly encouraged to lose weight (see Figure 1, p. 14). The good news is that losing 5–6 kg and moderate exercise is sufficient to restore ovulation in about half those affected, with many becoming pregnant with no further intervention. Even for women who do not become pregnant by themselves, this level of weight loss and exercise greatly improves the chance of becoming pregnant when fertility treatment is used.

As millions know from experience, losing weight and taking up exercise is not as easy as it sounds. Many fertility clinics arrange weight loss and exercise programmes where a small group of women in the same situation can support and encourage each other.

CASE HISTORY

Stella started her periods at age 13 and had regular periods until she went on the pill at age 17. She stayed on the pill until she was 32 and then stopped it in order to conceive. She was surprised that her periods did not return immediately and after six months (and many negative home pregnancy tests) she went to see her doctor. Her blood tests revealed that she had a high level of prolactin. Her specialist recommended a scan of her pituitary gland to rule out a large tumour. The scan was normal and Stella was started on bromocriptine. At first she felt slightly nauseated on the drug but gradually this passed. After six weeks of bromocriptine Stella had her first period. Her next period did not arrive, but this time it was because she was pregnant.

'Low-tech' interventions

Medication for hormonal imbalance

Ovulation problems can be due to hormonal imbalance and in many cases, this can be easily treated by medication. Overproduction of the pituitary hormone prolactin can inhibit the production of FSH and LH, the hormones responsible for ovulation. Bromocriptine is a specific drug that inhibits the secretion of prolactin. This oral medication is prescribed for women with high prolactin levels to restore normal ovulation. Fertility usually returns to normal allowing most women to conceive naturally.

Ovarian stimulation

Ovarian stimulation involves giving drugs to drive the ovaries. These range from tablets like Clomiphene citrate to injections of follicle stimulating hormone (FSH).

This treatment is very effective but the chance of multiple pregnancies (twins, triplets or higher multiple pregnancy) is very high if more than two follicles are stimulated to grow together. Limiting the number of follicles to just one or two is an art as much as a science.

The level of ovarian stimulation needs to be monitored using blood tests or ultrasound scans to limit the risk of multiple pregnancy. If there are too many follicles treatment is stopped and then restarted two or three weeks later at a slightly lower dose.

• **Clomiphene:** In addition to problems with being underweight or overweight, another cause of ovulation irregularities is polycystic ovary syndrome (PCOS), which prevents normal ovulation. This condition can be treated with medication. Clomiphene is a pill which is taken for five days in a row. It causes the pituitary gland to secrete more FSH which stimulates egg production and therefore induces ovulation.

There is a risk that Clomiphene may stimulate too many follicles, which increases the chance of twins, triplets or even greater multiple pregnancy. For this reason doctors take a cautious approach, starting with a low dose of Clomiphene and monitoring ovarian response using blood tests and usually an ultrasound scan. With this type of monitoring, the risk of multiple pregnancy is less than 9% of all births. During treatment you should have intercourse around the middle of the cycle or when an ultrasound shows there are appropriately sized follicles present. Clomiphene treatment is effective, with 30 to 50% of women conceiving within three to six months of treatment.

Clomiphene can also be used for another group of women: those who have regular periods but have unexplained infertility. No one knows exactly why it helps this group, but possible reasons are an increase in the number of follicles, and therefore eggs that are released each month, or better synchronising follicle development and hormonal preparation of the uterus.

The pregnancy rate in this group is more modest at around 15% per cycle, but still much higher than the 1 to 2% per month expected without treatment. Most of the pregnancies occur within the first four cycles of treatment.

• **Gonadotrophins:** Ovulatory drugs are used to prepare for fertility treatments such as in vitro fertilisation (IVF) and intrauterine insemination (IUI). These include drugs to increase the body's own

CASE HISTORY

Imogen had always had irregular periods. Her friends complained about their monthly painful periods whilst Imogen used to go for many months without a period, and then out of the blue she would have a heavy but pain-free period. Her doctor started her on the pill at age 16 'to sort her out'. Imogen stayed on the pill until she was 22. She then decided she wanted to take a break from the pill, as she was concerned that it had contributed to her weight gain. Her weight had slowly increased from 65 to 85 kg over the previous six years. When she discontinued the pill her periods stopped altogether and over the next year she noticed that her skin condition deteriorated with frequent outbreaks of pimples. She also became more hairy and grew a faint moustache along with increasing hair over the lower abdomen and nipples.

Imogen was referred to a gynaecologist, who performed blood tests and scans, which revealed the presence of polycystic ovaries. Imogen was advised to stay on the pill until she wished to conceive and to try to prevent further weight gain. Imogen's symptoms improved on the pill and she remained on it until she was 31. By this time she wished to start a family and so stopped her oral contraceptive.

After three months of no periods she saw a fertility doctor who started her on Clomiphene. Imogen did not respond to this drug and after six months of scans and blood tests she took a break and worked hard at getting fit and lost 4 kg.

On her next cycle of Clomiphene she conceived twins and delivered two healthy boys at 36 weeks.

level of FSH, or injections of FSH itself, so that the follicles are stimulated to produce eggs for fertilisation or to yield eggs that can be harvested. Gonadotrophins are also used in women who have failed to respond to the ovulatory drug Clomiphene.

Hormone treatment for men

Hormones like FSH can also be used for men with hormone deficiencies to try to increase sperm production. This is, however, a rare cause of male infertility and for most men with a lower-quality semen analysis there is no curative medication.

'Mid-tech' interventions

There are a couple of 'mid-tech' surgical or instrumental interventions which may be useful for select groups of patients.

Ovarian diathermy

Ovarian diathermy is a 'mid-tech' surgical operation to try to trigger ovulation in women who are not ovulating because of polycystic ovarian syndrome (PCOS), and who have not responded to Clomiphene. This procedure is done under general anaesthetic using laparoscopy. A laparoscope (telescope) and a diathermy probe are inserted through a small incision in the navel, and used to make small scars on the surface of the ovary using an electric current. This treatment is believed to act a bit like pressing the 'reset' button on a computer; the ovarian-pituitary hormone feedback is interrupted and restarts normally which induces ovulation and is successful in about 60% of women. It has a limited duration because most women stop ovulating a few months to a year after the procedure and eventually the ovary returns to its original PCOS condition.

Lipiodol flushing

Lipiodol flushing may be useful for women with mild endometriosis and possibly unexplained infertility. An iodine-based oil is pushed through the Fallopian tubes. Results from a small clinical trial showed that lipiodol flushing resulted in more pregnancies after three months than in women who did not have a flushing procedure. It is not known what mechanism may cause this.

Intrauterine insemination

Intrauterine insemination (IUI) is when sperm from your partner's

CASE HISTORY

Bruce runs a computer business and Helen is a teacher. They have had three years of unexplained infertility. All of Bruce's semen analyses have been normal. Helen's periods are regular and her hormone tests are normal. Helen's pelvis was entirely normal at laparoscopy. Bruce and Helen decided to try IUI with mild ovarian stimulation. Helen conceived on their second attempt and went on to have twins at 32 weeks. The twins are now five years old and, despite not using any contraception, they have not managed to conceive again. Bruce and Helen had another three cycles of IUI without success and now that Helen is aged 40 they have decided to stop all further treatment.

semen are placed inside the uterus using a catheter. It is a commonly used and relatively straightforward 'mid-tech' treatment that has the advantage of being moderately cheap and not too invasive. This procedure is used for several infertility problems, including:

- poor-quality mucus or mucus that is hostile to sperm, in order to bypass the cervical mucus
- unexplained infertility
- mild to moderate endometriosis
- mild to moderate sperm problems

IUI treatment is usually combined with mild ovarian stimulation using Clomiphene and/or low doses of FSH. Ovulation is monitored by daily blood tests around the middle of the cycle, or it can be triggered by hCG. The highly motile sperm in the ejaculate are isolated from semen in the laboratory and gently injected into the uterus around the time of ovulation. IUI is successful but does have limitations. One limitation is the risk of multiple pregnancy rate; it requires at least two or three follicles to achieve a reasonable pregnancy, and that means 15 to 20% of all pregnancies are twins and 1 to 2% triplets. A second limitation is the relatively modest pregnancy rate compared to IVF, typically 15 to 20% per cycle in women of 37 and younger. Nevertheless, three or four cycles of IUI can give an overall chance of pregnancy similar to that of a single cycle of IVF. Most pregnancies occur within the first four cycles of treatment. If a pregnancy has not occurred after four cycles, it is usually worthwhile considering moving to IVF.

'High-tech' interventions
In vitro fertilisation

In vitro fertilisation (IVF) is the process of adding together the egg and the sperm outside the woman's body so that fertilisation happens in the laboratory instead of in the Fallopian tubes. The early embryo development also takes place in the laboratory and once normal development is established the embryo is transferred back into the woman's uterus to continue its growth and development. IVF was first performed in 1978 and has since been successfully used to overcome infertility caused by a variety of factors, including:

- tubal disease
- endometriosis
- male infertility
- intractable ovulation problems
- unexplained infertility

As techniques have improved, the pregnancy rate from IVF has eclipsed that of all other types of fertility treatment.

Stage 1: Ovarian stimulation — The first stage of the IVF process is to ensure that there are sufficient numbers of eggs mature and ready for collection. The woman takes 'fertility drugs' to stimulate multiple ovarian follicles into maturing several eggs instead of just one. Six to 10 eggs is ideal; the more eggs the greater the chance of having a good-quality embryo to transfer into the uterus. However, this comes with a higher risk of complications such as ovarian hyperstimulation syndrome (OHSS), which varies from mild to severe with symptoms such as a feeling of bloating or abdominal pain.

There are various drug regimens for stimulating the ovaries. The most common and successful is to start by turning off the body's own reproductive hormones with the contraceptive pill and then use another type of drug, called a gonadotrophin analogue, so that there is more control over egg production. Next, FSH is given to stimulate the growth of several follicles in which the eggs develop. Follicle growth is monitored by blood tests and ultrasound scans every two or three days. Once the follicles reach the right size, final maturation of the egg is triggered by another hormone called hCG, and egg collection is timed for 36 hours later.

Stage 2: Egg collection — When the eggs are mature and ready for collection a needle is gently introduced through the vagina into the ovaries, using ultrasound to guide the needle into each follicle, and the egg is aspirated out of the follicle, along with the follicular fluid. This is repeated until all the mature eggs have been collected. At each collection the embryologist looks for an egg in the follicular fluid with the help of a microscope. The procedure usually takes about 15 minutes under local anaesthesia to help with relaxation and provide pain relief. The woman is awake and may have her partner alongside.

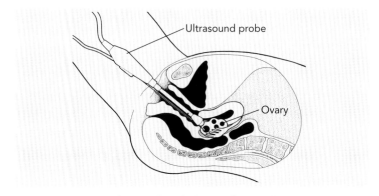

Figure 19: Ultrasound-guided egg collection showing the ultrasound probe close to the ovary.

Stage 3: Fertilisation — Over the next six hours, the embryology team prepare the partner's sperm and add this to the eggs. The eggs and sperm are left to mix in an incubator at body temperature for 14–18 hours. The next morning, the eggs are examined for signs of fertilisation, and the resulting embryos cultured for another three to five days in the laboratory under carefully controlled conditions.

Stage 4: Embryo transfer — The embryos are transferred into the uterus on days three to six. The best embryo is selected (or two for older women) and transferred into the uterus using a catheter inserted into the vagina. If there are several good-quality embryos, those remaining can be frozen for transfer at a later time offering another chance of pregnancy.

Embryo transfer is very simple and no more uncomfortable than having a cervical smear. It takes another nine to 11 days to know whether the embryo has implanted and started a pregnancy — which can be the longest days in many couples' lives.

CASE HISTORY

Cindy and Paul had been trying for a child for four years. Cindy was 34 and was feeling very despondent about their chances of ever having a child. All investigations were normal and so they were put into the 'unexplained' group. They became eligible for publicly funded treatment and on their second cycle of IUI with mild ovarian stimulation Cindy conceived. Sadly, she had a miscarriage at nine weeks. Cindy and Paul went on to have four further cycles of IUI without success. They were then advised to try IVF. Cindy responded well and produced eight eggs, of which six fertilised. One embryo was transferred and Cindy became pregnant and delivered her son eight months later.

Frozen embryos

Cryopreservation is the process of storing embryos, sperm and sometimes eggs in liquid nitrogen at very low temperatures, for later use. Using frozen embryos is a much simpler process than the stimulated IVF cycle. There are two approaches. Either the time of ovulation can be determined in a natural menstrual cycle from the results of daily blood tests, or hormonal drugs can be taken to create a controlled cycle. An embryo is thawed at the appropriate time and transferred into the uterus. About 70 to 80% of embryos survive the freezing and thawing process.

What are the chances of success with IVF?

The chance of success leading to pregnancy depends mainly on the age of the woman, as well as the quality of the egg and sperm. Because so many women now have only one embryo transferred at a time, choosing to freeze the rest, we commonly represent the chance of pregnancy per IVF cycle in terms of the percentage of pregnancies achieved for each IVF cycle, using the fresh embryo and then using frozen embryos if the first cycle (fresh embryo transfer) is unsuccessful.

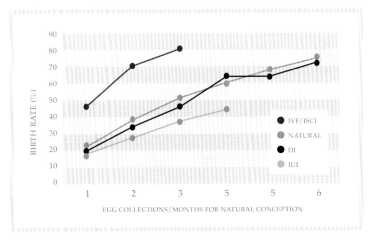

Figure 20: Cumulative pregnancy rates, 37 years and younger, at Fertility Associates for IVF treatment and donor insemination.

Variations on the IVF theme

The technology for assisted reproduction has advanced greatly over recent years and now there are some variations on the IVF theme to help couples become pregnant.

Intracytoplasmic sperm injection (ICSI)

ICSI is when a single sperm is injected directly into the egg to fertilise it. This technique is used when there is a serious sperm problem, including low sperm count, low sperm motility or the presence of sperm antibodies. If possible, sperm are isolated from the semen, but if not they are retrieved directly from the testes. ICSI is also used where there has been previous fertilisation failure with conventional IVF.

In conventional IVF around 50,000 sperm are placed with the eggs in the culture dish, which allows the fastest and most healthy sperm to fertilise the egg. If there are very few sperm or sperm quality is too low or uncertain, the injection of a single isolated sperm into each egg will maximise the chance of fertilisation. This technique means that IVF can be used for almost any type of male infertility as long as living sperm can

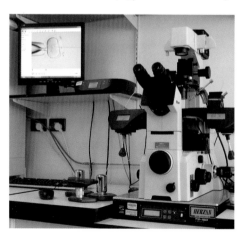

be found. Outcomes with ICSI are similar to those with IVF, apart from a slight increase in the number of children born with an abnormal number of X and Y chromosomes: 0.6% instead of 0.2% in the general population. Men whose infertility is genetic in origin may pass the condition on to their male children.

Above: The micro-manipulating microscope which is used to inject sperm inside an egg (intracytoplasmic sperm injection or ICSI).

Testicular sperm retrieval

There are several reasons for using the technique of testicular sperm retrieval, including:

- a blockage that prevents sperm from entering the ejaculate from the testis
- vasectomy
- so few sperm being made in the testis that they can not be found in the ejaculate

In these cases, sperm can usually be retrieved from the testis using a fine needle under local anaesthetic, and the retrieved sperm can then be frozen and used for ICSI at a later time.

Assisted hatching

Following embryo transfer, as part of the IVF procedure, the embryo has to 'hatch' out of its flexible 'shell', called the zona pellucida, and implant in the uterus, to initiate pregnancy. Assisted hatching involves making a small hole in the zona pellucida just before embryo transfer, to make it easier for the embryo to hatch and implant. Some studies indicate assisted hatching is helpful, others do not: it may be more helpful in increasing the chances of successful implantation using frozen embryos, and particularly in older women.

Blastocyst culture

The blastocyst is the name for the embryo when it is around five days old and has begun to specialise. Blastocyst culture involves growing the embryo in the laboratory for longer than the usual three days until it has matured to the blastocyst stage and then transferring it at around day five after egg collection, instead of day three. Blastocyst culture offers the possibility of a higher pregnancy rate from the fresh embryo transfer due to better embryo selection.

Many embryos, whether they arise naturally or after IVF, have chromosomal abnormalities that we cannot easily detect. These abnormalities stop the embryo from developing much beyond the eight-cell stage which occurs on day three. With blastocyst culture, embryologists can choose embryos on the basis of their ability to develop, rather than their physical appearance at an early stage.

Studies show blastocyst culture can increase the initial pregnancy rate, but not the overall pregnancy rate, when the subsequent use of any frozen embryos is considered. Because only around 30% of all embryos develop to the blastocyst stage, some couples will have no blastocysts to transfer by waiting the extra few days.

Our approach at Fertility Associates is to focus on choosing the best embryo for fresh transfer. Sometimes blastocyst culture is the best way of achieving that goal; sometimes the best embryo is already apparent by day three before reaching the blastocyst stage.

Egg freezing

Egg freezing is when the eggs are frozen soon after egg collection instead of having sperm added to them. Egg freezing may be a useful option when no sperm are available during an IVF cycle, if a couple feels uncomfortable with having 'spare' embryos frozen, or where a single woman wishes to preserve her fertility prior to cancer treatments or possibly for social reasons. Egg freezing is a much newer technology and success rates are more difficult to estimate.

Preimplantation genetic diagnosis

Preimplantation genetic diagnosis (PGD) involves analysing embryos for genetic abnormalities before they are transferred, to detect any chromosomal abnormalities or inherited genetic diseases. The technique involves removal of one or two cells from an eight-cell embryo at day three after fertilisation. An opening is created in the zona pellucida using a laser and the cells are removed using a small suction pipette. The cells are then analysed using one of two molecular biology techniques:

• Polymerase chain reaction (PCR) — in which fragments of DNA (genetic material on the chromosomes) are amplified, so that it is possible to look for a known genetic mutation which causes diseases such as cystic fibrosis, muscular dystrophy or Huntington's disease.

- Fluorescent in-situ hybridisation (FISH) — in which fluorescent chemicals, called probes, bind to specific chromosomes so that the tagged chromosomes can be visualised under a fluorescent microscope. It is possible to count the number of each chromosome and so detect the presence of common chromosome problems, such as Down syndrome (Trisomy 21).

The results from PGD are available within two days and the unaffected embryo(s) can then be transferred to the uterus as a blastocyst(s) on day five. The major application of PGD is to prevent the conception and birth of children with genetic abnormalities, particularly in families carrying serious inherited genetic conditions. Recent consensus is that the present level of PGD technology does not increase pregnancy rates when applied to IVF or ICSI when used to treat infertility.

Fallopian tube surgery for women

When to choose Fallopian tube surgery

For some types of damage to the Fallopian tubes, surgery may offer a similar chance of success as IVF. In addition to surgery to restore fertility, it is sometimes recommended before IVF to increase the chance of success.

When surgery is a possibility, the decision between IVF and surgery requires careful assessment by a doctor who has expertise in both fertility and surgery. The decision must take into account the type of damage, risk of ectopic pregnancy and the age of the woman. The woman will usually require a diagnostic investigation, such as laparoscopy or ultrasound, to assess the degree and type of damage before this decision can be made.

Hydrosalpinges

Damaged Fallopian tubes can cause fluid accumulation making the tubes swell up. These swollen fluid-filled tubes are known as hydrosalpinges and can be seen by ultrasound. Hydrosalpinges reduce the chance of IVF pregnancy probably by secreting fluid into the uterus which interferes with implantation. The removal of hydrosalpinges by surgery can double the chance of pregnancy with IVF.

Sterilisation reversal

Surgery is often the best option for reversal of sterilisation. In the last decade most female sterilisations have involved clips on the Fallopian tubes. If the tubes have not been damaged too much, surgery offers an 80% chance of pregnancy in women aged 38 or younger at the time of reversal.

What is involved in Fallopian tube surgery?

The surgery itself is performed using a laparoscope or a small incision in the abdomen. In some circumstances, an operating microscope is needed for the careful dissection and repair of damaged tissue. This is time-consuming and delicate work that requires extensive training in microsurgical techniques.

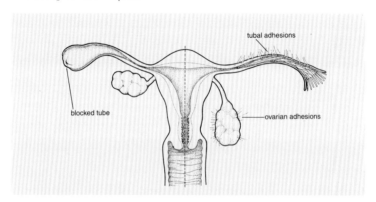

Figure 21: Different types of operations which may be performed on damaged Fallopian tubes.

Advantages and disadvantages

Surgery has both advantages and disadvantages. If successful and you become pregnant after surgery, then there is every chance you will be able to become pregnant again and therefore surgery is a solution that offers the opportunity of a family not just a single pregnancy, unlike a

CASE HISTORY

At age 36 with two children, Dan had a vasectomy. At 45 he found himself in a new relationship with Laura, aged 32. She wished to have a child and so Dan underwent a vasectomy reversal. Sadly, no sperm were present in the ejaculate after the reversal so they then struggled with their options. These included another attempt at the reversal operation, an IVF-ICSI cycle in which sperm would be extracted from the testes, or the use of donor sperm. They decided to try IVF-ICSI treatment. Laura conceived and subsequently delivered a daughter. Laura and Dan do not wish to have any further fertility treatment.

single cycle of IVF. Also, there is no need for treatment with hormones or other fertility drugs before surgery and the process is quicker. For older women, surgery is particularly advantageous as it offers a chance at pregnancy every month, even if the chance per month is low. On the other hand, the disadvantage of surgery is an increased risk of ectopic pregnancy, which is typically 10% following surgery.

Surgery for men

Vasectomy reversal

Generally the only fertility surgery performed on men is vasectomy reversal, since surgery in other circumstances is rarely useful. Rejoining the two cut ends of the vas deferens is technically difficult because of its small size and its many blood vessels. For this reason it should be undertaken by a highly trained microsurgeon.

Even when technically successful, vasectomy reversal may not restore fertility because the immune system makes antibodies against sperm. Antibodies can interfere with the way sperm swim through the woman's cervical mucus and can block fertilisation. About 50% of men who have a vasectomy reversal father a child without further intervention, although this depends on the number of years between the vasectomy and its reversal. It is not uncommon for sperm to reappear in the ejaculate after reversal but later, after a year or more, to disappear again due to scarring at the site of the operation.

Varicocele surgery

One controversial area of male surgery is operating on the varicoceles, small varicose veins in the blood supply to the testes. Although they are more common in men experiencing infertility, they are also very common (incidence of around 15%) in men without any fertility problems. How they might influence fertility is still debated, a possibility is that varicoceles may raise the temperature of the testes slightly. Research shows that the combination of smoking and a varicocele is particularly bad for fertility. Most well-designed studies have failed to show any advantage to surgically repairing varicoceles.

Using donors for assisted fertility treatment

So far we have considered making the most of a couple's own sperm and eggs through various fertility treatments. However, sometimes there are situations where donor sperm or donor eggs are a logical consideration, including:

- a man has no sperm
- a woman has been through menopause
- pregnancy has not occurred despite repeated IVF treatments and the fertility potential of the man's sperm or the woman's eggs is questioned
- single women or women in same sex relationships

Donor legislation

Donor treatment and surrogacy (described below) come with important social and ethical responsibilities, and all are highly regulated in New Zealand to look after the interests of the children, the donors and surrogates as well as the couple or single woman who wants a family. Some types of donor treatment are 'established procedures' under the Human Assisted Reproductive Technology (HART) Act which means they are available 'off the shelf'. A few require case-by-case application to the national Ethics Committee on Assisted Reproductive Technology (ECART). ECART applications are always needed for surrogacy, embryo donation, and sperm or egg donation between

CASE HISTORY

Jack and Sarah are farmers and are both in their early thirties. They had been trying for a pregnancy for two and a half years and came to Fertility Associates to check whether anything was wrong. Sarah had regular periods and had no past history of any problems. Her hormone tests were normal. However, Jack's sperm analysis showed only two million sperm per millilitre (the usual count is over 20 million). He gave no history of problems with his testes but noted that he had been exposed to the usual farm chemicals, pesticides and herbicides.

The options we discussed included donor insemination or an IVF and ICSI cycle. Jack and Sarah saw a counsellor in order to help them decide which treatment option was right for them. Initially they decided on ICSI treatment but as two cycles were not successful and because of the distance and expense involved they decided to change to donor insemination. After three cycles of donor insemination, Sarah became pregnant. They have elected to store their donor's sperm for more children in the future.

family members who are not brothers, sisters or cousins. An example would be a mother donating eggs to her daughter.

For sperm and eggs donated after August 2005, donors must be identifiable. Under the HART Act the clinics notify the Department of Births, Deaths and Marriages whenever a child is born using donor sperm, donor eggs, or donor embryos donated after August 2005, or when a child is born after surrogacy. Births, Deaths and Marriages hold basic identifying information about the donor that can be accessed anytime after birth by the parents or by the child when he or she reaches adulthood. The clinics offer the same service, with the addition of counselling to help prepare people for exchanging information.

Donor sperm

Donor sperm is used where a man has no viable sperm and by single women or same sex couples, who often try self-insemination at home, turning to a clinic if this does not work. Donors may be recruited by fertility clinics or personally by the recipient. The process of sperm

CASE HISTORY

Sue and Debs had been in a relationship for some years when they decided they would like to have a child. Debs decided that she would be the one to become pregnant. They approached a fertility clinic, where Debs had an examination and some blood tests. They went to counselling and then took their time to select a donor. Eventually they used a known donor. He was carefully screened for infectious diseases such as HIV and hepatitis B. His semen was frozen for three months and then treatment was started. Debs had a regular cycle. Blood tests showed her LH surge, which meant that she could then go into the clinic for the insemination. After three cycles of treatment, Debs had not conceived. She underwent a laparoscopy, which showed a few tiny spots of endometriosis, which were removed. Debs became pregnant after the next cycle of donor insemination. Their child is now two years old and Debs is undergoing treatment again.

donation involves the following stages:

- The donors are screened for their family medical history and for diseases than can be transmitted through semen.
- Sperm is frozen and typically banked over several months for its future use.
- Three to six months later the screening tests are repeated, and the frozen sperm can be made available for use.
- Counselling is essential for both the recipient and donor, and covers the implications of being a donor or having children conceived in this way.

How donor sperm is used depends on the quality and quantity of the banked sperm, the age of the woman, and the presence of any other fertility factors. The simplest approach is IUI without ovarian stimulation, with insemination timed by blood tests. Adding mild ovarian stimulation increases the chance of pregnancy especially in older women. If sperm quality is lower, or the amount of sperm available is limited, or IUI has not worked, then the donor sperm can be used with IVF or even ICSI.

For younger women, the chance of pregnancy from simple IUI with

CASE HISTORY

Beth was treated for Hodgkin's disease at age 21. Her chemotherapy and radiotherapy cured her disease but made her ovaries fail and so she became menopausal. Five years later, Beth and Pete decided to have a child. Beth's older sister, Louise, offered to donate her eggs.

After careful counselling, Louise came through an IVF cycle and produced six eggs, which were donated to Beth and Pete. Four eggs fertilised normally but a pregnancy did not result and Louise had found the process very stressful. Two frozen embryos were replaced but once again no pregnancy resulted.

Beth had another cycle of egg donation using an altruistic donor recruited by the clinic. They met Jane prior to the cycle as Beth and Pete wanted any children they would have to know about the origin of their genes and how special they were. Jane produced 14 eggs and 10 fertilised. One embryo was transferred and Beth became pregnant and had a healthy baby. A further five embryos have been frozen and Beth and Pete hope that their daughter may have a brother or a sister some day. Beth and Jane keep in touch once or twice a year and plan to continue to do this.

donor sperm is about 20% per month, similar to that of fertile couples (see Figure 20).

Donor eggs

Donor eggs are used for two broad scenarios, lack of eggs or poor-quality eggs.

Lack of eggs can be caused by early menopause or no response to ovarian stimulation for previous IVF treatment which has therefore been unsuccessful. Many women who do not respond to IVF drugs will be peri-menopausal and enter the menopause within the next five years or so.

Poor quality eggs may be the problem either because of a woman's age or because she has not become pregnant after several IVF cycles and this can reduce the chance of success of conventional IVF.

The process of egg donation involves the following stages:

- The donor undergoes the steps of IVF stimulation up to and including egg collection.
- The eggs are then donated to the recipient couple and fertilised with the recipient partner's sperm.
- The recipient woman also receives hormonal drugs to synchronise her 'cycle' so that her uterus is at the right stage to receive the transferred embryo.
- Again counselling is essential, as the donor also has to be prepared for the medical risks of IVF.

In New Zealand about half of all donor egg cycles involve a close friend or family member as the egg donor. Pregnancy rates are similar to that of conventional IVF, but depend on the donor's age rather than the age of the recipient.

Donor embryo
Couples who have completed their family but still have frozen embryos remaining have the option of donating those embryos to another couple or woman. This treatment is technically simple; the recipient woman's menstrual cycle is monitored with daily blood tests and an embryo is thawed and transferred at the right time. Complexity arises because the recipient's child, if there is a pregnancy, will be a full sibling of the donors' children. ECART requires separate and joint counselling for those involved, and a police check of the recipients as in adoption.

Surrogacy
There is also the option of surrogacy for women who no longer have a uterus or for whom carrying a pregnancy is too risky to their health.

Surrogacy involves a woman having a baby for another couple. In simple surrogacy, the surrogate mother is inseminated with sperm from the commissioning couple, and so the child is biologically hers to the same degree as her own children. Fertility clinics are involved in IVF surrogacy, where the commissioning couple provide the embryo after

CASE HISTORY

Diana had cancer of the cervix at age 27 and needed a hysterectomy. She had no children. When she was 30, Diana was given the all clear in terms of her cancer and then she and her partner began to talk about the possibility of having a child. Diana's ovaries were not removed and a check of her hormones revealed that she was producing eggs normally. Diana's sister, Christine, had had three children and offered to be Diana's surrogate. They are now involved in counselling and hope that they will be able to have a cycle of IVF surrogacy later this year.

undertaking all the IVF steps themselves, apart from embryo transfer. Surrogacy requires extensive separate and joint counselling for all involved. A surrogacy agreement is drawn up by lawyers acting for each party as well as approval from ECART. Nevertheless, the woman who carries and gives birth to the child is still the legal mother, and the commissioning couple need to adopt the child. The adoption process needs to be pre-approved by Child, Youth and Family (a service of the Ministry for Social Development) before treatment starts.

What about alternative therapies?

There is a lot that Western medicine doesn't know so some alternative therapists may have some useful options. We are often asked what options we would recommend, ranging from Chinese herbs, aromatherapy, naturopathy, reflexology, osteopathy and acupuncture. The only alternative therapy that has been subjected to a number of well-designed studies is acupuncture. A recent review found that women who had acupuncture at the time their embryos were replaced in an IVF cycle were more likely to get pregnant compared to women who did not have acupuncture.

We would also like you to stop alternative therapies whilst you are having fertility treatments, except for acupuncture. Chinese herbs are drugs in their natural state, and many have not been tested for their effect on hormone production, sperm, eggs or embryos and may have a negative impact.

CHAPTER EIGHT

PREGNANCY

For couples fortunate enough to have become pregnant this chapter provides some information about preparing for the arrival of your baby and some problems to be aware of.

How do you know when you are pregnant?

Most women know they are pregnant because of those tell-tale signs like suddenly feeling tired or nauseated and developing sore breasts. The most obvious sign that you are pregnant is a late period, particularly if you are used to having regular monthly cycles. By the time four days have gone by after you should have had a period, you may well be pregnant. However, an unusual period that is perhaps shorter or lighter than a normal period is not uncommon in early pregnancy. In fact about one-third of women experience some bleeding in early pregnancy, either in the first few weeks or around the time when their period would normally occur. If you suspect you are pregnant, the best confirmation is a pregnancy test.

Pregnancy tests

A pregnancy test measures the amount of the hormone human chorionic gonadotrophin (hCG) in the blood or urine. This hormone is secreted by the developing embryo and its placenta and can be detected as early as 10 days after conception, which means you can be tested as soon as you have missed a period. Measurement of hCG in blood is more accurate and will give an exact level, whereas urine testing can be done using a pregnancy testing kit that you can buy from your pharmacy or supermarket. If you are pregnant you will usually test positive on the first day of the missed period; however, beware of false positives and always read the instructions carefully.

What causes those early signs of pregnancy?

Common symptoms of pregnancy are tiredness, nausea, breast tenderness, increased urinary frequency, moodiness and headaches. Most women experience some of these symptoms in early pregnancy, and whilst for many women they are a minor inconvenience, for a few they may be overwhelming, necessitating bed rest or occasionally hospital admission.

• **Tiredness:** The feeling of extreme tiredness and lethargy in early pregnancy may be enormous, making it very difficult to carry out the simplest tasks. Most women start to feel better around 12 weeks of pregnancy although for some women this tiredness lasts throughout their pregnancy. The exact reason behind this tiredness is not known, but presumably it relates to the huge physiological and metabolic changes occurring during this time.

• **Nausea and vomiting:** These are classic symptoms of early pregnancy and affect most but not all women. Commonly known as 'morning sickness' because symptoms are supposedly worse early in the day, for many women the feelings of nausea last all day and are often worse when tired, such as early evening. Eating regular small quantities of food usually helps. The nausea is thought to be related to the increasing amounts of pregnancy hormones being produced by the placenta. A twin pregnancy can cause more severe nausea due to higher levels of these hormones. Once again, the problem usually improves after 12 weeks, although for some unlucky women it may persist throughout the pregnancy.

• **Appetite changes:** This is very common in pregnancy. Many women go off tea and coffee in early pregnancy, whilst others do not fancy red meat. Some become ravenously hungry, while others develop a metallic taste in the mouth, usually associated with increased saliva production. These food-related changes are again probably associated with changes in your physiology, such as digestion, taste and sense of smell, and in some cases your body is telling you what it needs.

• **Breast changes:** In early pregnancy most women experience breast changes, which may be a feeling of heat, enlargement, tingling or indeed pain, as the breast tissue changes and prepares for milk production.

• **Frequent urination:** The need to pass urine more frequently in early pregnancy is caused by the increased amount of fluid in your body and increased blood flow to the kidneys, which make more urine. Also, pressure on the bladder as the uterus expands can make this worse.

• **Mood changes:** Some women experience mood changes, which can be either uplifting or depressive in the early months, possibly caused by an increased blood flow through the brain.

Antenatal care
Options for antenatal care
Changes in maternity benefit legislation have altered the antenatal choices for women in New Zealand. Currently, you may have free antenatal care by a midwife or GP (many GPs have given up obstetrics because of the new funding changes) or you may see a specialist through the local maternity hospital. Alternatively, you can see a specialist privately. The cost for private care varies enormously and may range from a few hundred to over four thousand dollars. It is best to phone and ask.

When to see a specialist
Many GPs and specialists work with independent midwives, allowing further options. Whether you need a specialist depends on your pregnancy. If you have a medical problem or pregnancy problems, including previous obstetric problems, a multiple pregnancy or you are pregnant following IVF treatment, you should definitely see a specialist during pregnancy. If you develop a problem during pregnancy or delivery, your lead maternity carer (LMC) may arrange a consultation with a specialist.

When to start antenatal care
You will probably have your first antenatal visit at around 12 weeks. However, if you have had a previous miscarriage or ectopic pregnancy or you wish to discuss prenatal diagnosis, an earlier visit is advisable.

What are your dietary needs when pregnant?

Maintaining a balanced diet is usually all that is required during pregnancy. Make sure you eat lots of fresh fruit and vegetables and cut down on processed foods. However, there are some dietary changes you should make and some things to watch out for. which are listed in the following table:

REQUIREMENTS FOR A BALANCED DIET

Folic acid: Having enough folic acid is important in pregnancy, as it minimises the chances of having a baby with neural tube defect (spina bifida). It is found in most plant foods, especially green leafy vegetables, wholegrain breads, cereals and legumes (peas, beans and lentils). However, it is important to take folic acid tablets to make sure your intake is sufficient (0.8 mg per day until 12 weeks of pregnancy). Also, folic acid combined with a general multivitamin such as Elevit has been found to reduce heart, urinary tract and cleft lip abnormalities.

Vitamin A: Although vitamin A is important for normal development, high doses have been shown to be harmful in early pregnancy and can cause birth defects. Fruit and vegetables (particularly yellow vegetables like carrots) are a good natural source of vitamin A. Vitamin A supplements should not exceed 10,000 IU (international units) and high vitamin A-containing foods, such as liver, should probably be avoided in pregnancy.

Iron: A reasonable dietary intake of iron is needed during pregnancy. The best source of iron is red meat. If you don't eat much red meat, you may need an iron supplement. You should discuss this with your caregiver.

Calcium: Pregnancy imposes considerable calcium demands and if you don't eat dairy products then you may need to take calcium supplements. Another good source of calcium is sardines.

Iodine: It is also important to have a reasonable intake of iodine, as it is important for thyroid hormones which are needed for normal development of your baby. You can get sufficient iodine from iodised salt.

Listeria: This is a common bacteria present in soil, water, plants and sometimes in human and animal faeces. Good hygiene in food preparation is very important in pregnancy, to prevent contamination with listeria. Most of us are exposed to listeria frequently without ill effects; however, occasionally it can cause miscarriage or stillbirth. The most common foods that may contain listeria are cheeses made from unpasteurised milk, pre-cooked chicken, ham and other pre-cooked meat products, stored salads and coleslaws, and chilled pre-cooked seafood products.

What is prenatal diagnosis and what tests are available?

There are a number of tests available that may help determine whether your baby has any problems prior to birth. The problems that these tests can detect include:

• **Chromosomal abnormalities:** This usually means the wrong number of chromosomes (too many or too few), for example Down syndrome, which is caused by an extra number 21 chromosome. Abnormalities can also be caused by a structural defect where chromosomes become broken or rearranged. Chromosomal abnormalities usually happen during cell division in the maturing egg or in the early embryo and may lead to a variety of problems in the baby, including structural abnormalities, severe mental retardation and infertility. This can happen in any pregnancy but is more common with advancing maternal age (see Table 3), following the previous birth of a baby with a chromosomal abnormality or where either parent is known to carry a chromosomal problem.

• **Some inherited diseases:** These are where a malfunctioning gene is passed on from parent to child. Examples of inherited diseases include Huntington's disease, haemophilia and cystic fibrosis, which are caused by a gene mutation on a specific chromosome. Where a family history is present, it is important to identify these genetic problems as they can be passed on to your children.

• **Anatomical defects:** The most common are neural tube defects, which occur in three out of every 1000 pregnancies and include problems such as spina bifida or anencephaly (where the baby's brain does not develop properly). Folic acid supplements can significantly help to reduce this risk.

Amniocentesis

Amniocentesis is the most common procedure used for diagnosing genetic abnormalities. A small amount of fluid is removed from the amniotic sac surrounding the baby, through a fine needle that is inserted through the wall of the uterus, guided by ultrasound. This amniotic fluid contains cells and proteins from the baby. The cells can be used to identify chromosomal abnormalities and some inherited diseases. A particular protein, alpha-fetoprotein fluid, is analysed to detect spina bifida. Amniocentesis cannot reliably be performed before 14 to 16 weeks of pregnancy and there is a risk of 0.5% of causing a miscarriage. Results may take two weeks to be available, although in some cases results may be ready within two or three days in some centres (where newer technology is available) which exclude the most common abnormalities. It is important to weigh up all factors before having amniocentesis, as you may have to make the difficult decision of whether or not to have a termination.

Chorionic villus sampling (CVS)

This procedure also identifies chromosomal abnormalities and can be done earlier than amniocentesis, usually at 11 to 13 weeks of pregnancy. Again a fine needle is inserted through the abdominal wall and a small sample removed; in this case a biopsy of the developing placenta is taken. For this procedure, the risk of miscarriage is about 0.5 to 1% and, as with amniocentesis, initial results can be available within two or three days but the complete result takes two weeks.

Ultrasound

This is a scanning procedure, which is done at around 18 weeks of pregnancy. Many women choose to have an ultrasound as this has been shown, with increasing accuracy, to determine whether the baby has any anatomical abnormalities. There is no evidence that ultrasound is harmful to mother or baby.

Nuchal fold ultrasound

Many ultrasound units are now offering nuchal fold ultrasound. This type of ultrasound scan measures the neck fold thickness of the baby at 12 to 14 weeks of pregnancy. Studies have found this to be an accurate but not absolute determinant of chromosomal problems, such as Down syndrome, where the measurements are greater than in an unaffected baby. While it carries no risk to the pregnancy, it only provides a risk estimate of likelihood of chromosomal abnormality, unlike amniocentesis and CVS, which provide certainty about outcome rather than an assessment of risk. Sometimes a nuchal fold assessment may be combined with a blood test from the mother to give a more accurate risk of chromosomal abnormality.

New techniques

Researchers continue to improve techniques to separate out fetal cells that can be collected from the maternal blood and the mucus in the cervix. It may be possible that in the near future a blood test from the mother or a cervical smear could determine the exact chromosomal make-up of the baby, from which abnormalities can be identified.

Problems in early pregnancy

Bleeding

About one-third of women experience some bleeding during early pregnancy. Sometimes it is an indicator of miscarriage but usually it is not. You should contact your doctor or midwife if you are having bleeding, so that you can be given an examination and scan. Rest is also usually advised, although it is unknown whether this has any influence on the outcome of the pregnancy.

Hyperemesis

This is an extreme form of morning sickness, where severe vomiting and nausea prevent adequate intake of food and liquid. Whilst many women feel nauseated or may sometimes vomit in early pregnancy, a few women cannot tolerate any food or fluids and can become dehydrated and malnourished. Often intravenous fluids will be needed and a scan should be performed to exclude multiple pregnancies or other rarer problems. Thyroid function tests should also be performed, to check that there is no problem with production of thyroid hormones.

Ectopic pregnancy

Ectopic pregnancies occur when the embryo implants in a site other than the uterus. The most common site is in the Fallopian tube, but human embryos have also been known to grow in the cervix, the ovary, the liver and the lining of the abdominal cavity. As the embryo begins to grow there is a risk that a blood vessel may burst, causing internal bleeding. Ectopic pregnancies occur in about one in 200 pregnancies, and may even occur following IVF treatment, but are more likely in women with damaged tubes or in women who have had previous ectopic pregnancies.

Typical symptoms include lower abdominal pain, vaginal bleeding and, rarely, faintness. The diagnosis of an ectopic pregnancy may be difficult, and is usually made with a combination of examination findings, ultrasound, pregnancy hormone levels in the blood and sometimes laparoscopy. Unfortunately, there is no way of moving an ectopic pregnancy into the uterus so that it can continue on to become a viable pregnancy. The treatment for an ectopic pregnancy is removal of the pregnancy using surgery or sometimes with drugs.

Pregnancy after fertility treatments

Pregnancies after fertility treatments have the same risk of miscarriage as pregnancies conceived without medical intervention. An early ultrasound (around seven weeks) is recommended to make sure that the pregnancy is viable and has implanted normally in the uterus. An early ultrasound will also determine the number of embryos present. There is a slightly increased risk of fetal growth problems following fertility treatments and therefore specialist care is generally recommended.

Pregnancy in older women

The modern trend is for women to have their babies later in life, as contraception has become more reliable and careers more important. It used to be thought that pregnancy in the over 35-year-old woman carried a much increased risk but modern data would definitely not support this view. The chance of miscarriage or having a baby with a genetic problem such as Down syndrome does increase with increasing age (see Table 3) because of a reduction in egg quality. However, other pregnancy-related problems do not increase with age.

Some medical problems such as diabetes and high blood pressure may occur more frequently as a woman gets older, so it would be wise to have a general check before trying to get pregnant.

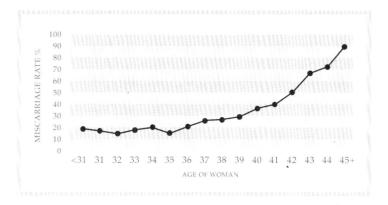

Figure 22: Chance of pregnancy loss by maternal age.
(From ANZARD data published mid 2008.)

AGE	RISK OF ABNORMALITY	AGE	RISK OF ABNORMALITY
20	1:2000	42	1:26
30	1:800	43	1:20
35	1:172	44	1:15
36	1:74	45	1:11
38	1:66	46	1:7
39	1:54	47	1:7
40	1:44	48	1:7
41	1:35		

Table 3: Chromosomal abnormalities at 16/40 weeks' gestation according to maternal age.

CHAPTER NINE

MISCARRIAGE

It is very common to lose a baby by miscarriage early on in a pregnancy. In fact about 15% of all confirmed pregnancies end in miscarriage and this is known because pregnancy testing is now so sensitive that it is possible to confirm that you are pregnant in the very early stages. This means that a miscarriage can also be recognised earlier. Over 90% of all miscarriages happen within the first 12 weeks of pregnancy.

What are the signs of a miscarriage?

Very early miscarriage

A miscarriage can happen as early as five weeks into the pregnancy, probably before you even know you are pregnant and it is more like a late and heavy period. This is known as a 'biochemical' pregnancy because you start to produce pregnancy hormones but the embryo does not survive long enough to develop into a recognisable fetus which can be seen on an ultrasound scan.

First trimester

If you know you are pregnant, then the first warning sign of a miscarriage is heavy bleeding that does not stop and low, cramping, period-like pains. Although as many as 30% of all normal pregnancies do have slight bleeding within the first three months, you may suspect there is a problem as you might suddenly stop feeling pregnant. For example, you might lose some of the symptoms you have had, such as nausea and vomiting, which, unpleasant as they may be, are reassuring signs of a normal healthy pregnancy.

After three months

Losing a baby after 13 weeks can actually be like going into labour. Your waters may break and you may feel contractions, just like being in labour.

What causes a miscarriage?

Most miscarriages are unavoidable as the developing fetus could never become a normal baby. This is either because something has gone wrong in the early stages of its development or because of inherited chromosomal abnormalities. There are also other factors that increase the chance of miscarriage, especially for women who have repeated miscarriages. These are:

Maternal age

All the eggs you will produce throughout your life are already with you at birth and they age as you do. The chance of an egg being abnormal rapidly rises as you age (see Figure 22), especially over the age of 35 years, as older eggs have more chromosome abnormalities, which increases the risk of miscarriage. The average age of women getting pregnant for the first time is increasing in New Zealand, which means that miscarriage is becoming a more common problem.

Genetic causes

You or your partner may be a carrier for an abnormal chromosome that does not affect your health but may be lethal if inherited by your baby. Inherited tendencies to miscarriage on both sides of the family may also predispose to miscarriage, as does your own health as a baby.

The phospholipid syndrome

Antibodies are normally produced as part of the body's immune defence, but there are a group of antibodies, produced against a substance called cardiolipin, which is a phospholipid and is a normal part of the body's cells. They do not affect the mother's health however, they may attack and damage the fetus in its early stages as the embryo implants into the uterus; also the placenta may come under attack later in pregnancy. So having these antibodies in your blood may predispose to miscarriage in early and late pregnancy.

Uterine problems

A weak (incompetent) cervix may open too early and cause a miscarriage in the later stages of pregnancy (often 14 to 20 weeks). Other structural problems with the uterus that may cause a miscarriage include irregular shape and the presence of a dividing wall of tissue or scar tissue, as these may interfere with normal fetal development. Fibroids (benign growths), especially if they are small, are unlikely to be a cause of miscarriage.

Infection

Some infections at a critical stage of pregnancy can cause miscarriage. Those that have been implicated are rubella, toxoplasmosis and cytomegalovirus, although any infection that causes a high temperature can cause problems.

Hormone problems

If the ovary does not produce enough progesterone (the hormone produced during the later phase of the menstrual cycle which maintains the lining of the uterus in case an egg is fertilised), this is called the 'defective luteal phase' and may be a potential cause of miscarriage, although this is still a controversial area.

Recurrent miscarriage

Because miscarriage is so common, some couples will, by chance alone, experience the problem more than once. If you have had three or more miscarriages you should seek referral to a specialist for investigation into the cause.

It is likely, however, that no specific cause will be found in at least half of all couples who have had three miscarriages. Recurrent miscarriage is a very distressing experience as couples who have had this problem require not only full investigations of their problems but also more intensive antenatal care in the first part of the pregnancy. Some hospitals run early pregnancy clinics to see women with a history of miscarriage more frequently in the first three months of pregnancy. With supportive care of this kind, 80% of women with a history of recurrent miscarriage will have a continuing pregnancy and live baby.

What should you do if you think you are having a miscarriage?

If you start bleeding early in your pregnancy, you should always visit your doctor or midwife for a check-up and to try to identify the cause.

Here are some of the investigations you will need to help decide whether you are having a miscarriage and whether or not you are at risk of losing your baby.

Ultrasound scan

Your developing fetus can be seen as early as five weeks using an ultrasound scan and at six weeks you will be able to see its tiny heart beating, which is a very reassuring sign, especially if you have been bleeding before you are 10 weeks pregnant. A visible heartbeat means that you have a 95% chance of keeping your baby. Even if bleeding continues or starts after 10 weeks there is still an 85% chance that your pregnancy will continue.

If a heartbeat cannot be seen there may be other explanations. For example, you may have your dates wrong and your pregnancy may be earlier than you thought (a good reason to record dates of periods and to note ovulation times when trying to conceive), or your uterus may be in a position that hides the fetal heart. Often a vaginal scan will give a more accurate picture of how an early pregnancy is progressing. This is where the probe is placed in the vagina.

Because changes and growth of the fetus in the first three months of pregnancy are so rapid and dramatic, it is possible to see whether development is as it should be. Therefore a scan is usually repeated after one to two weeks. This will usually help your doctor decide very clearly whether or not the pregnancy is progressing normally.

Blood tests

You may also need blood tests to help confirm what the ultrasound shows, particularly early on in the pregnancy when it is too early to see a heartbeat on a scan. Blood levels of the hormone hCG double every two to three days between four and six weeks of gestation. If you are at risk of a miscarriage, monitoring this hormone in your blood can provide a good indication of the well-being of your pregnancy.

What next?

If your fetus is alive and well and all the indications are good then there is no clear evidence that there is anything you can do to ward off a miscarriage. If your developing fetus is abnormal nothing will prevent nature from taking its course and miscarrying the pregnancy.

Look after your body

Your lifestyle can make a great difference to the well-being of your pregnancy. Evidence from women who have had repeated miscarriages indicates that rest is important and that activities such as prolonged standing, lifting and shift work should be avoided. Any 'toxin' that you take into your body may affect your baby and therefore you should not smoke or drink alcohol and you should limit your coffee intake.

Don't feel guilty

You must not feel guilty that it was something you did that contributed to the miscarriage. You may think it was because you had sexual intercourse or went travelling during your pregnancy you lost your baby, but these will not cause a miscarriage. It is most likely that your baby was already lost and that the cause of the bleeding, whether it was the act of sexual intercourse or another activity, was just the trigger for the miscarriage that would have happened anyway.

What happens if miscarriage is inevitable?

If a miscarriage is inevitable because your baby has already died, you do have a choice as to how you handle the miscarriage, but you should always discuss options with your doctor or midwife to help you decide which is best for you.

- You can await a spontaneous miscarriage, which means that you will bleed and the pregnancy will be shed, in a way similar to a heavy period.
- You can have the pregnancy tissues removed surgically by a procedure called an evacuation of the uterus.
- Another option is to take medication called misoprostol that induces the lining of your womb to be shed, along with the pregnancy. Misoprostal is not currently registered for use in New Zealand.

If you are prepared to wait for the miscarriage to happen naturally, then you will probably not need an evacuation, which is true for 80% of early miscarriages. You should always keep a close watch for signs of infection and a follow-up ultrasound scan is needed to make sure the uterus is empty. If you still need an evacuation because of infection or because you have heavy or continuing bleeding, this can sometimes be done under a local anaesthetic.

Allow yourself to grieve

No matter at what stage of pregnancy a miscarriage happens, it is still the loss of a baby and often a much longed-for baby. The grief that you feel can be just as severe as losing a baby after it is born. Everyone's experience is different. For some women it is possible to accept the miscarriage after quite a short period of time; for others changes in emotions and behaviour may be experienced over a long period. These feelings may include:

- fear of being alone
- loss of confidence and self-esteem
- their body has let them down
- anger and disappointment with partners, medical attendants, family and friends
- hostility to other pregnant women
- tendency for food and drink binges

If you have feelings like these it is a time to seek help from understanding friends, family, health professionals and the local miscarriage support group.

It is also important to know what has happened to the baby. Although it is not usually possible to recognise a 'baby' in the tissues obtained from the uterus when an evacuation is performed early in pregnancy, you may want to take the tissues home for a private burial, but if they are left at the hospital they are cremated separately and with respect.

Often parents wish to know why the miscarriage occurred. This is only possible to find out by a chromosomal analysis, as the usual hospital examination cannot tell if the baby is abnormal or not. However, this analysis is usually only arranged under special circumstances.

Here are some commonly used terms and their meanings:

• **Abortion:** An outdated term for miscarriage; it is still occasionally used but does not imply that anything was done to cause the miscarriage.

• **Threatened miscarriage:** There is bleeding in early pregnancy but the cervix is closed and the pregnancy is still alive, or it is too early to be sure from ultrasound scanning if the development is normal.

• **Inevitable miscarriage:** There is bleeding present and the cervix is opening.

• **Blighted ovum:** There may be normal symptoms of pregnancy and the pregnancy may carry on for several weeks or months. When a scan is done only the placenta and membranes can be seen as the embryo has either failed to develop or has been reabsorbed very early on in the pregnancy. This is also sometimes known as an empty sac.

CHAPTER TEN

SURVIVING AND LIVING WITH INFERTILITY

'Give me children or else I die'
Genesis, Chapter 1, Verse 13

Rachel's words from Genesis highlight the depth and intensity of the emotional agony that commonly accompanies the experience of infertility. This experience involves many losses that have to be weathered, usually without any preparation and with limited understanding or support from the general community. This may make infertility a very lonely and isolating experience.

This chapter will discuss the impact of infertility on a couple's life and how to develop strategies for coping with these issues.

How does infertility make you feel?

Many people grow up with an expectation that they will be able to have children whenever they wish. If this does not happen a whole range of emotions can be triggered, including a significant loss of confidence.

As one woman put it:

'If I can't do the simple feminine thing that all women are meant to be able to do, how can I do anything? My life's plan was that I would grow up and have children. I feel cheated that the road for me is different and no one told me that this could be. I wonder what else might lie in wait for me.'

One man said:

'Every time someone at work celebrates his wife having a baby I think, "What sort of man do they think I am?" '

Creating a new life, especially with a chosen partner, is a unique event. Losing this opportunity and with it a genetic interest in the future and links with generations in the past, can leave a gap, or emptiness, which for most people is devastating and is felt throughout their lives.

No children means no grandchildren.

'Who will want to fondle my treasures and look through the family photos when I die, remembering me in the process?'

'My cat is a reluctant recipient of all the love I have to give, but I can't read it bedtime stories and enjoy watching it travel through life's transitions. Never will I be able to experience my child's first day of school, her triumphs, her sorrows.'

Coping with emotions and stress
Loss of control

Feelings of failure and a loss of self-confidence, together with a declining feeling of optimism about the future, can bring about a very debilitating sense of loss of control and loss of choice. Those people who choose, voluntarily, not to have children have exercised their choice and can feel satisfied they are in control of their lives. In contrast, infertility removes the choice people believed they had. It is well documented that people who have little control over their lives may experience feelings of hopelessness and helplessness and that these feelings can, over time, bring about a state of clinical depression.

Why can't I fix it?

Just imagine trying month in and month out, year in, year out to achieve a pregnancy. You give up alcohol and coffee; you pray, hope, think positively, exercise (but not overly strenuous exercise), and do all the things you know you should to prepare your body. You are still not pregnant and soon feel that no matter what you do you cannot control your fertility.

We are all so used to problem solving by planning and then implementing those plans; in other words, fixing problems by doing something. This also applies to fertility problems, and when it comes to trying to overcome infertility, you will commonly experience great frustration and feelings of helplessness.

Are you obsessed?

Having difficultly conceiving can mean 'getting pregnant' becomes the most important goal in life. The intense desire to continue pursuing this goal and the depth of the pain experienced on this journey is often underestimated by the couple themselves. Worse still, they may be dismissed or labelled by family and friends as desperate or obsessed. But the fact is that infertility affects every aspect of a person's life. It permeates through all domains — the sexual relationship, friendships with fertile friends, family relationships, career plans, holiday plans, and financial plans; all of life's plans.

Little wonder then that infertility can have a dominating influence in a person's life. It is just not possible to 'forget trying to get pregnant and get on with other things', or 'relax, and not think about it', advice that people experiencing infertility find hurtful and lacking in understanding.

Couples experiencing infertility long for it not to dominate their lives and invade every discussion about future plans. But just as parents have to consider their children every day, so too do childless couples have to plan around their childlessness.

Changing relationships

Sexual relations with your partner

As you strive to achieve a pregnancy, sex often becomes a means to an end with the continual hope that 'this may be the month'. The failure to meet this goal has to be confronted month after month. Relationships are bound to change, as investigations into the causes and medical assistance to become pregnant only add to the sense that sex can no longer be private, spontaneous and enjoyed for its own pleasure. Enduring many years of infertility often leaves a permanent scar on a couple's sexual relationship.

'It felt so mechanical, it was horrible; I don't want our sexual relationship to be like that. We comforted ourselves with the knowledge that we had probably "done it" at the right time and therefore it was a chance taken.'

Another couple commented, 'We have given up on our sexual relationship. We always ended up fighting around ovulation time with the pressure of having to perform, so we gave up even trying. The idea of having sex for pleasure seems a distant memory.'

Almost all couples experience negative changes in their sexual relationship, and seeking advice from a professional may remedy losses in this area.

Friends and family

Not only do sexual relationships suffer, so too can relationships with friends and often family members. Being surrounded by pregnant friends, hearing about relatives' pending births and observing the excitement, joy and sense of achievement that is often generated by the arrival of a new family member only exacerbates the losses that you will be feeling. There are no flowers, fusses or presents for you; only the sad thoughts, 'Why not us too?' 'When will it be me?' 'It should be our turn!'

Talking about infertility with friends and family may not be easy either. Who can you tell? Because many couples see their infertility problems as a private matter, they don't tell anyone and thus deal with their grief within the relationship. This is a lot to ask of each other and commonly one partner may have a desire to talk to close friends or family but will not do so in order to protect the other partner.

It may be too difficult to explain to friends and family, no matter how close, that envy and jealousy are part of how an infertile person feels, especially if the response is likely to be judgmental rather than compas-sionate. Consequently communication is often censored, the closeness enjoyed in relationships may be lost and friends may drift apart.

Relationships can survive!

Friendships with people who are good listeners, who help explore and verbalise feelings and experiences without judging, are likely to survive and can be a valuable source of support. Those people who do share some of their journey with others usually find it a relief to 'come out of the closet'. As one man put it:

'I can't believe I kept my infertility a secret for four years; the more I put off telling my parents, the harder it became and the more fearful I became of them finding out that our child was conceived with the help of a donor. I became obsessed with protecting the secret to the great detriment of my emotional health, my work and my relationship with my wife. Now that I have told them I feel a huge burden has lifted off my shoulders.'

Others keep close friends in touch from the beginning.

'I couldn't imagine not being able to talk and sometimes cry about our infertility. It's the only way I can stay sane about it. I'm lucky, I have one good friend who just listens, lets me cry and doesn't try to analyse my experience or cheer me up with other people's miracle stories.'

Looking for the reason

Finding a reason for infertility is emotionally helpful. Although it may be hard to face at the time, an early diagnosis, if possible, is an aid to taking control and offers an opportunity to make decisions about treatment options, or future life plans.

If there is a definite diagnosis of azoospermia (absence of sperm in the semen) or blocked Fallopian tubes, then wasting years of precious time trying and hoping, which is also emotionally detrimental, could be avoided. Therefore, seeking a diagnosis is a step towards emotional equilibrium.

These statements are almost guaranteed to exacerbate emotional distress:

'Wait and see', 'Wait another six months', 'Don't worry; you're young, there's plenty of time to worry later.'

If no cause can be established for a couple's infertility this can deliver a double blow, as expressed by this sentiment:

'Not only am I not pregnant, I can't explain why. Maybe it's my punishment for my past. Perhaps it's all in my head!'

However, finding the cause brings its own losses. These include loss of dignity, loss of privacy and a sense of personal invasion:

'I'm usually a confident, assertive woman used to coping but when I come to the clinic I feel like a transparent jelly that could be pushed over and just go splat. It's not that the staff treat me badly — they're wonderful — I just feel vulnerable.'

Treatment also brings stress. The merry-go-round of raised hopes and expectations, and the disappointment, devastation, even depression following treatment that doesn't work is emotionally draining. It takes a toll on even the most optimistic and expert stress manager.

However, deciding to embark on infertility treatment means at last you can exercise some control and 'do something' that increases your chances of conceiving:

'On our third IVF cycle I was losing hope and energy to keep trying, but now I'm so grateful we persevered for our dream of having our family finally came true.'

Coping strategies

Surviving infertility is a challenge that requires a 'multifaceted' approach. Here are some coping strategies:

• **Seek information and become informed about options:** This is one way to increase the feeling of control. Good sources of information and support are available through Fertility New Zealand and the Miscarriage Support Group. Their newsletters keep people in touch with what's happening and where.

• **Find support groups:** These are run by the societies and are probably one of the most useful resources; here you can meet others in the same boat and can talk openly, knowing that others will truly understand the depth of your pain and the dilemmas you face.

• **Seek counselling:** Seeing a counsellor who specialises in infertility early on in the journey can be very useful in helping people to access resources and options, as well as giving them the opportunity to discuss and explore the impact that infertility is having on them.

Seeking counselling, however, is very difficult for people who feel they should be able to cope on their own.

In their words!

No one writes about infertility better than people who have been through it:

'We wish we had gone to see the counsellor when we first found out rather than struggle on pretending we were all right. It was such a relief to be able to talk with someone who could help us see things from a different perspective. We came away feeling reassured that we weren't going crazy after all; we were grieving. Knowing that has allowed us to express our grief rather than bottle it up until we explode. We now accept that our grief comes and goes. The journey is a bit like a roller coaster; sometimes it's easier to cope with than others.

We now plan for the result on the months we have treatment, and try to have another focus with each monthly cycle. It's been important to channel our creativity into other areas. Creating and developing our garden, doing cooking and art classes has given us a lot of fun and pride and made us realise that just because we haven't been able to create a baby, it doesn't mean we aren't creative people.'

'Infertility has been the hardest knock I've ever had to face. I feel incomplete; my family is incomplete. I'm left with a huge hole that, no matter what other diversions I try to fill it with, will always be there. Nothing seems worthwhile or fulfilling.'

'I'm on a journey. I thought I knew what the route was. It's as if the roads are closed and there aren't any other paths to take.'

'If only someone could have told me that one day we would

definitely have children, even though not biologically from both of us, it would have helped guide me through the long painful journey. But when well-meaning friends and family used to say "You'll have children — I just know it", I used to feel so angry. They couldn't possibly "know" I'd have children — how could they? No one, even the doctors, could tell me that. And it's not knowing that is probably one of the hardest things to cope with. But now all that uncertainty is over. I look at my precious children with wonder, I certainly don't take them for granted and often remind myself how lucky we are to be parents.'

For those not so lucky, this last statement captures the experience:

'We'll always live with infertility as a backdrop to our lives. What I can say is that it is no longer centre-stage and no longer demands my full attention.'

Glossary

Amniotic membrane: Inner membrane around the amniotic fluid containing a fetus.

Anencephaly: Severe neural tube defect in which there is no brain development.

Anovulation: Lack of ovulation.

Anti-Müllerian hormone (AMH): A hormone produced by the small follicles in the ovaries. AMH can be measured in a blood test and is used as a marker of ovarian reserve.

Basal body temperature: Body temperature when you first wake up before undertaking any physical activity. Ovulation leads to increased progesterone levels, which are associated with a small rise in basal body temperature.

Blastocyst: Embryo five days after fertilisation, contains around 100 cells which have specialised into two distinct layers; one develops into the fetus and the other into the placenta.

Body mass index (BMI): Measure of body mass determined by dividing your weight (in kg) by height (in m^2). Normal values are between 20 and 25. Values of 30 or more are considered obese.

Chlamydia: A sexually transmitted bacterial infection that may damage the reproductive system.

Chorionic membrane: The outer layer of the membranes that surround the fetal sac.

Chromosome: Structures in the cell nucleus that contain our hereditary material (genes) in the form of DNA.

Cilia: Minute hair-like projections that line some tubes, e.g., the Fallopian tubes.

Corpus luteum: A yellow structure in the ovary that is formed after the rupture of the egg from the follicle producing progesterone.

Cryptorchidism: Undescended testes.

Dilatation and curettage (D & C): Operation to scrape out the lining of the uterus — also called an evacuation.

Dyspareunia: Pain during sex.

Ectopic pregnancy: Implantation of the fetus outside the uterus, commonly in the Fallopian tube.

Ejaculate: The discharge of semen from the penis during male orgasm.

Endometriosis: The presence of endometrial tissue at sites outside the lining of the uterus.

Endometrium: Lining of the uterus.

Epididymis: A gland sitting on the surface of the testis comprising tightly coiled tubes in which sperm are stored and mature in after being produced by the testes.

Ethics Committee on Assisted Reproductive Technology (ECART): This is a government appointed ethics committee which approves applications for surrogacy, embryo donation and certain instances of egg or sperm donation on a case-by-case basis.

Fallopian tubes: Two tubes that run from the uterus out towards each ovary that transport the egg towards the uterus and also help the passage of sperm.

Fecundity: The probability of a live birth from one cycle of ovulation.

Fetus: The developing baby in the uterus.

Fibroid: Benign muscular growth in the uterus.

Fimbria: Delicate, finger-like fringes at the ends of each Fallopian tube, that collect the egg and guide it into the tube.

Follicle: A fluid-filled sac in the ovary in which the egg matures.

Follicle stimulation hormone (FSH): A hormone produced by the pituitary gland that stimulates eggs to mature. FSH levels rise as menopause approaches.

Follicular phase: The first half of the menstrual cycle in which the dominant follicle grows to reach maturity, completed at the time of egg release (ovulation).

Gestation: Length of pregnancy.

Granulosa cells: Cells that surround each egg and line each follicle that are responsible for providing the egg with nutrients and producing oestrogen.

Human chorionic gonadotrophin (hCG): A hormone produced by the developing placenta that stimulates the corpus luteum to continue progesterone production so that the uterine lining remains and menstruation does not occur.

Infertility: Infertility is defined as the failure to conceive after one year of regular, unprotected sex.

Intracytoplasmic sperm injection (ICSI): Technique used for severe male infertility problems in which sperm are injected into eggs using a high-powered microscope.

In vitro fertilisation (IVF): The reproductive technique in which fertilisation occurs 'in vitro', which means 'in glass', i.e., in the laboratory. The resulting embryos are then transferred into the uterus to develop normally.

Laparoscopy: Technique in which a telescope visualises the structures within the abdomen. Commonly used to check tubal patency and to remove endometriosis.

LMP: Last menstrual period.

Luteal phase: The phase of the menstrual cycle from ovulation to the start of the next period.

Luteinising hormone (LH): A hormone produced by the pituitary gland that initiates the onset of ovulation.

Menarche: Onset of menstruation.

Menstruation period: The lining of the uterus is shed as a consequence of falling oestrogen and progesterone levels at the end of the luteal phase of the menstrual cycle.

Oestrogen: A hormone produced by the ovaries, which prepares the uterus in the first half of the menstrual cycle.

Ovary: The female gonad that contains the eggs.

Ovulation: Release of the egg from the ovary.

Pelvic inflammatory disease: Infection of the Fallopian tubes and uterus, which can lead to infertility by adhesion or scar formation.

Peri-menopause: The five to 10 years prior to cessation of periods (menopause).

Phyto-oestrogens: Oestrogens in plants.

Pituitary gland: A small gland at the base of the brain that produces FSH, LH and other hormones.

Placenta: The organ that transfers nutrients and oxygen from the mother to the baby.

Progesterone: A hormone produced by the corpus luteum, that prepares the uterus for pregnancy in the second half of the menstrual cycle.

Pronuclei: Once an egg has been fertilised, two pronuclei may be seen, one containing chromosomes from the egg and one containing chromosomes from the sperm.

Puberty: The time in adolescence in which sexual organs mature and secondary sexual characteristics appear.

Scrotum: The pouch that contains the testicles.

Spermatogenesis: Sperm production.

Spermatogonia: The cells within the testis that differentiate into sperm.

Spina bifida: A developmental abnormality in which the spinal cord is exposed.

Subfertility: A less than normal capacity for reproduction. Subfertility means that pregnancy is possible but the chances have been reduced due to a variety of possible reasons.

Testes: The male gonads responsible for production of sperm and testosterone.

Ultrasound: High-frequency sound waves that may be used to identify structures of the body.

Zona pellucida: Outer covering or 'shell' of the egg.

Useful contacts

Fertility New Zealand
Head Office, PO Box 12049, Beckenham, Christchurch 8242
Phone   Support Line 0800 333 306
                Administration Line 09 332 7790
Email   us@fertilitynz.org.nz
Website   www.fertilitynz.org.nz

Miscarriage Support Group
PO Box 147 011, Ponsonby, Auckland 1144
Phone   Support Line 09 378 4060
                Administration Line 09 360 4034
Email   support@miscarriagesupport.org.nz
Website   www.miscarriagesupport.org.nz

Recurrent Pregnancy Loss Clinic
Fertility Plus, Greenlane Clinical Centre
214 Greenlane West Road, Greenlane, Auckland 1051
Phone   09 630 9988
Fax   09 631 0728
Website   www.adhb.govt.nz

New Zealand Multiple Births Association
PO Box 1258, Wellington 6140
Phone   0800 489 467
Website   www.nzmba.info

New Zealand Endometriosis Foundation Inc.
PO Box 1673, Christchurch Mail Centre, Christchurch 8140
Phone   Support Line 0800 733 277
                Administration Line 03 379 7959
Fax   03 379 7969
Email   nzendo@xtra.co.nz
Website   www.nzendo.co.nz

FERTILITY ASSOCIATES
Phone 0800 10 28 28
www.fertilityassociates.co.nz

Auckland
Level 3, 7 Ellerslie Racecourse Drive,
Remuera 1051
Private Bag 28910, Remuera 1541
Phone   09 520 9520
Fax   09 520 9521
Email   faa@fertilityassociates.co.nz

Auckland North Shore
Apollo Centre for Health and
Wellbeing
Level 1, 119 Apollo Drive
Albany 0632
Phone   09 477 3676
Fax   09 477 3777
Email   fas@fertilityassociates.co.nz

Hamilton
Level 2, 62 Tristram Street,
Hamilton 3204
PO Box 598, Hamilton 3240
Phone   07 839 2603
Fax   07 839 2604
Email   fah@fertilityassociates.co.nz

Palmerston North
2/22 Victoria Avenue
Palmerston North 4410
Phone   06 354 5537
Fax   06 354 7781
Email   faw@fertilityassociates.co.nz

Wellington
Level 2, 205 Victoria Street,
Wellington 6011
PO Box 11048, Manners Street,
Wellington 6142
Phone   04 384 8401
Fax   04 384 8402
Email   faw@fertilityassociates.co.nz

Whangarei
Whangarei Area Hospital
Hospital Road, Whangarei 0110
Phone   0800 10 28 28
Email   faa@fertilityassociates.co.nz

Tauranga
Promed House, Suite 9
71 Tenth Ave, Tauranga 3110
Phone   0800 10 28 28
Email   fah@fertilityassociates.co.nz

Rotorua
Lakes Care Medical Centre
1165 Tutanekai St, Rotorua 3010
Phone   0800 10 28 28
Email   faw@fertilityassociates.co.nz

Hawkes Bay
The Royston Centre
325 Prospect Rd, Hastings 4122
Phone   0800 10 28 28
Email   faw@fertilityassociates.co.nz

Gisborne
8 Fitzherbert St, Gisborne 4010
Phone   0800 10 28 28
Email   faw@fertilityassociates.co.nz

Nelson
132 Health Centre,
132 Collingwood Street,
Nelson 7010
Phone   0800 10 28 28
Email   faw@fertilityassociates.co.nz

PUBLIC PROVIDERS OF FERTILITY TREATMENT

All Fertility Associates clinics are public providers of fertility treatment; however the following organisations also offer public treatment.

Fertility Plus
Private Bag 92189, Auckland 1142
Phone   09 630 9810
Fax   09 631 0728
Email   carolo@adhb.govt.nz
Website www.adhb.govt.nz

Otago Fertility Services
Dunedin Hospital, Private Bag 1921, Dunedin 9054
Phone   03 474 7752
Fax   03 474 7690
Email   fertility.services@healthotago.co.nz
Website www.healthotago.co.nz

The Fertility Centre
Hiatt Chambers, First Floor, 249 Papanui Road, Christchurch 8146
Phone   0800 433 784
                      03 375 4000
Fax   03 355 8851
Email   info@nzcrm.co.nz
Website www.nzcrm.co.nz/christchurch

Index